Books by Beth Alderman

THE EVOLVE FERTILITY SERIES

BOOK 1
Melissa's Match: *Great Society*
ISBN: 978-1-7321110-1-1

BOOK 2
Connie's Conception: *Awareness of Peril*
ISBN: 978-1-7321110-0-4

BOOK 3
Melissa's Malady: *End of Modernity*
ISBN: 978-1-7321110-2-8

BOOK 4
Colette's Creativity: *Sacred and Profane*
ISBN: 978-1-7321110-3-5

BOOK 5
Colette's Community: *Thirds*
ISBN: 978-1-7321110-4-2

CHRONIC ILLNESS OWNER'S MANUALS

*Regenerate Your Life: Chronic Illness as a Springboard
for Creating Your Best Life*
VOLUME ONE: ISBN: 978-1-7321110-8-0
VOLUME TWO: ISBN: 978-1-7321110-9-7

MEANINGFUL RETIREMENT:

Become a Life Care Provider
ISBN: 978-1-7332849-0-5

EVERYWHERE FOREVER

*What To Do When Ubiquitous
Artificial Toxins Disable You*
ISBN: 978-1-7332849-6-7

BOOKS BY BETH ALDERMAN

THE EVOLVE RESTORATION SERIES
Sequel to the Evolve Fertility Series

BOOK 1
Pilgrim Minds: *After the War on Life*
ISBN: 978-1-7321110-5-9

BOOK 2
Aaron's Legacy: *The Body of Life*
ISBN: 978-1-7321110-6-6

BOOK 3
The Kindred's Rebirth: *Rough Seas and Far Lands*
ISBN: 978-1-7332849-3-6

BOOK 4
Jacki's Vision - Part One: *The Green Line*
ISBN: 978-1-7332849-4-3

Jacki's Vision - Part Two: *Ethos*
ISBN: 978-1-7332849-7-4

BOOK 5
Mel's Motherhood: *A Place in the Living World*
ISBN: 978-1-7332849-5-0

Everywhere
FOREVER

WHAT TO DO WHEN UBIQUITOUS
ARTIFICIAL TOXINS DISABLE YOU

Beth Alderman, MD, MPH

FUTURE MEDICINE LLC • ASHLAND, OREGON

Everywhere Forever
What To Do When Ubiquitous
Artificial Toxins Disable You

By Beth Alderman, MD, MPH
© 2025 Future Medicine LLC
www.LivingFutureBooks.com

Book Design: BookSavvyStudio.com

ISBN: 978-1-7332849-6-7 (paperback)

First Edition
Printed in the United States of America

To Dr. Fernando Vega

and

*In memory of the doctors of the
Essex Scottish Regiment*

Contents

Next morning, we started for [Wales]. On this tour I had a striking instance how easy it is to overlook phenomena, however conspicuous, before they have been observed by anyone. We spent many hours in Cwm Idwal, examining all the rocks with extreme care [b]ut neither of us saw a trace of the wonderful glacial phenomena around us; [a] house burnt down by fire did not tell its story more plainly than did this valley. If it had still been filled by a glacier, the phenomena would have been less distinct than they now are.

— CHARLES DARWIN

[Hansen] knew that PCBs, for example, were mass-produced for years before studies how's that they accumulate in the food chain and cause a range of health issues, including damage to the brain. This most reliable way to gauge the safety of chemicals is to study them over time, in animals and, if possible, in humans. What Hansen didn't know was the 3M had already conducted animal studies—two decades earlier. They had shown PFOS to be toxic, yet the results remained secret, even to many at the company.

— SHARON LERNER in *'You Make Me Sick'* in *The New Yorker* 5/27/24

A Note to You

AFTER 2,500 YEARS, THE ART OF MEDICINE IS NO MORE. Drowned in molecularism, and strangled by information systems, it is regrettably no longer available to us as we navigate the challenges of the Sixth Extinction.

Responsibility for personal and planetary healing now falls on the shoulders of we who are sick. As we care for our bodies and lives by means offered in my books and developing websites, we can revive medical naturalism, grasp new-to-evolution ailments caused by modern humans, recover our inborn abilities, and protect life from the core of our bodies. It is up to us to 'put on our own oxygen masks first' and learn to navigate the new dangers that threaten us and imperil life on earth.

In this book I share my memoir as an academic physician epidemiologist and patient disabled by one of the new insidious epidemics that medical specialists are observing like the blind ment with the elephant who saw only the one part of the problem they could touch. I had dedicated my working life to getting to the bottom of new epidemics, and when I was disabled, stepped off the treadmill of modern ways of acting, and fell back on the lost ancient tradition of medical natural history, I was able to reverse the toxicity that threatened my body and my life.

You can see how to use medical naturalism to save your own lifetime. In Everywhere Forever, I recount my use of the ancient medical art of defining an actionable problem and solving it. This process is not precise, but unlike the new 'precision medicine' medical naturalism is valid and accurate and effective. And, it provides a roadmap for you to follow as you face the unprecedented human-caused ailments that others cannot yet see because no technology can do this for you. Thinking is required.

As we do our chosen part to reconcile human crimes against creation, and so to restore a living future we can recognize that the stakes are no less that taking advantage of a once in eternity chance to save evolution. Because our sun is already middle aged, evolution has no time to start again from a world without forests, which will soon be a world with oxygen. Should we fail to help ourselves with the habitats that give us life, the learning encoded in your DNA may disappear, and the next big bang may never again supply the conditions for evolution.

The good news is that humans now know all that we need to do to solve our present predicament, and to take this chance to regard nature with unceasing love, wonder and gratitude that we are always free to accept and reciprocate. Then, through the ancient path of suffering, we can become fully human and learn to live in harmony with the life on earth that gives us life.

Please accept the gift of my blood, sweat, and tears and pay it forward with your own gifts to care for your body and cure your life. When you are recovering, and better able to appreciate the fierce grace of illness that has given you this precious opportunity to rescue your life, you will be better able to appreciate your body and life.

With well-wishes, blessings, and the hope that you will find words in this book that will encourage you to curate your own knowledge, your wise actions, and your agency for the restoration of life from your core,

BETH ALDERMAN, MD, MPH
Ashland OR 2025
Living Future Books, LLC

EVERYWHERE

FOREVER

CHAPTER ONE

Falling into Shadow

———————

DECEMBER 1996. The only thing I knew to do was to push, to try harder. "I can't" was very difficult to get to. It took nearly a decade.

That makes sense. I am a soldier's daughter and a doctor. The way I was raised, and the way doctors are trained, there is no "can't." As military children, we keep at it, or die trying. As doctors in this age of modernity and automation, we keep trying until our databases tell us there is nothing left to try.

The moment of the crash wasn't when my symptoms started, or when my decline began. It was the day I finally collapsed.

That day began like any other, with a tense race to stay on schedule. My physician husband had risen at five. By five-thirty he was peddling up our gravel drive on his bike in the rain. After a twenty-minute ride in the dark on hilly, winding roads, he would spend forty minutes on the ferry to Seattle followed by half an hour on the bus to the hospital where he worked. I was up by six getting myself and the children ready for our respective days. After making sure they were dressed and had eaten breakfast, their lunches were packed, and their backpacks contained whatever was needed, I would drive my eight-year-old son to primary school and my three-year-old daughter to family day care. He was all business; she was all play and a love bunny.

As we dashed through the morning, I could feel the usual inner battle raging between the careerist and the mother inside me. The mother in me wanted to slow down, to relish these moments with my children; to be more nurturing, less driven and driving. As usual, the careerist won. She had to, if I was going to sustain the life I had signed up for.

I had a demanding and fulfilling career as an epidemiologist and professor. By definition, that required me to suppress my homebody maternal side and resist the pull of the nest. This had been going on since my son's birth—the yang professor bullying the yin homemaker, and prevailing. Ultimately, my heart's needs and wants came last. They ended up in the attic with the keepsakes, put off for some other, more opportune time.

Bundling my children into their rain gear and then into the car, I gave myself the oh-so-familiar talking-to, the one that kept me on the path my husband and I had worked so hard to earn and had begun with such determination. By nine, I was finally sitting at my computer in our cozy study off the living room, a fire in the high-efficiency wood stove burning behind me. This was my moment to focus. I sipped a cup of tea and tried to relax as I prepared to work. Outside, the rain had stopped. The fir trees, ferns, and rhododendrons were dripping, and a weak sun was penetrating the mist. I was alone in the sticks, aware that I was lucky to be able to telecommute, and to cut back on my hours again and again as the mysterious symptoms that had plagued me since my first pregnancy gradually took over my life.

I sighed deeply. I switched on my computer. I opened the manila folder I had left beside it the day before and reviewed my notes. I pushed aside any thought of my many nagging ailments. As the computer booted up, I turned my focus to its blank screen.

I had trained in public health and preventive medicine, and had become a medical detective. My life purpose was to find out what caused illness, and how to prevent it or cure it before it became irreversible. In my academic jobs, I researched the causes of problems in pregnancy, especially birth defects. That morning, I was preparing to analyze new data from my study of clubfoot.

I was looking at how it developed in utero, and whether it was a deformation (where tissue initially develops normally), or a malformation (where cells or tissues have a structural problem from the start). If it was a deformation—e.g. the result of pressure due to a lack of supporting amniotic fluid, or a uterine fibroid pushing the foot and misshaping it—then defects like it might have similar causes and could be grouped together for study and prevention. That would move the field of birth defects research closer to prevention because it would classify cases by cause as well as consequence, and might contribute to early detection and prevention of clubfoot.

I was excited about the work, and about being on the verge of analyzing data from my big five-year study. I felt close to an important discovery.

But that morning, I couldn't seem to get started. It didn't help that the statistical modeling methods, though state-of-the-art, were simple-minded. Biology is complicated, and my work involved visualizing a complex causal web, which pushed the limits of understanding. I had already identified the many plausible events that might lead to clubfoot. I had a sense of how they all fit together, and I had drawn it out on paper. I should have grasped all the details easily.

But that day, the events seemed like a cluster of marbles scattering in all directions, and I couldn't seem to follow any one of them. Order was lacking. I simply could not gather the elements in my mind. I couldn't analyze the data either. I knew it all by heart, but the longer I sat there, the more my mental circuits seemed to short and burn out. My heart sank.

No! I barked in silent command to my brain. *NO, not NOW! I'm so close!*

Nothing. I rubbed my scalp. I went for more caffeine, refilling my cup with strong black tea. I stretched. I walked in circles, trudging slowly, trying to get blood flowing all the way to the top of my head. I went back to my workstation and waited patiently for my inner fog to clear.

It didn't.

At noon I stopped for lunch. I microwaved one of the cheap frozen burritos that I ate to save money, then had an apple so that my diet wouldn't be too unhealthy. I shook breakfast crumbs off one of our place mats and positioned my plate and glass on it. I sat down. I took a bite of the burrito. Perfect. Chewing and swallowing—with difficulty; my esophagus just didn't seem to work right—I began to feel some hope. Sometimes food made a huge difference. Maybe the afternoon's work session would go better. I certainly hoped so.

As I ate, I looked at a picture of my kids hanging on the wall of our country kitchen. My daughter sitting like a little princess in her first dressy dress, my son kneeling sweetly beside her. I thought about the parents who were worrying about their unborn children. They were relying on me and others like me to know what to do. These were my working hours—but I had nothing to show for a whole morning's work. And I was getting paid. If I had been stronger, healthier, more vital, I would have panicked. But I didn't have the energy. Apparently guilt was a more accessible feeling, because the guilt in that moment was overwhelming.

I looked at the forest outside, which was recovering from long-ago clear cutting for the construction of tall ships, followed by strawberry farming, and took heart from its resilience. I had also tried to keep up the moldy house by painting the interior. Perhaps I, too, would make a new start after lunch. I brewed a cup of green tea as a tonic and took it back to my workstation.

I didn't recover after lunch. I sat in that chair all day. I stared at the screen. I tried to focus. I willed myself to focus. I could not work—and I could no longer ignore the fact that my own illness needed my attention. My work focused on a problem that was well-studied and relatively tractable. My own was daunting. It was wholly mysterious, and I knew it. I had pinpointed things that made my symptoms better or worse, but had failed to trace them back to causes. No one I knew could help me with that, and now I was losing the ability to help myself. I willed my fingers to move across the keyboard. I willed my brain to register what I was seeing on the screen, to make sense of it. I looked at my notes. Nothing. I looked back at the screen. Nothing. Hour after hour. Nothing happened.

It was as if the biggest part of me was still asleep. Nothing penetrated that wall of fog. Nothing slipped past it. My fingers could have moved, but nothing came from the brain for them to type. I didn't lose track of time; it wasn't that kind of fog. It was the kind of fog where you know you are asleep and every minute is a struggle to wake up into clarity. I couldn't do it.

In the past decade, I had pushed on through gastritis, depression, asthma and allergies, mysterious rashes, aches, pains, endless viruses, and flus that never seemed to go away. I had struggled with unreliable childcare, with working in a sick building, and with helping aging parents.

But today's mental paralysis was crippling. It was a show stopper. No analysis, no work. No work, no vocation. And no meeting expectations—mine, my research unit's, my patients', or society's. Until that moment, my life had felt possible. I could believe in the value of hard work. I could believe in the values of the system that I had grown up in, been trained in, and adhered to. More than that, I could believe in myself, that I could do this, and that it was worth doing.

Sometime around four that afternoon, I knew it was over. All of it.

"I can't … " I said softly to myself. "I just … can't."

I sat there for some time, feeling the urgency of my effort ebb away from my body. With it went what little strength I had left.

This scared me. I was finally, truly, on empty.

I relaxed. I let go. There was nothing for it.

And that's when it finally happened.

The crash. The failure of my willpower, my tolerance, and my adrenal overload. My symptoms broke through like a red alert, and I couldn't believe that I hadn't felt them before. I fell into a hell of pain and suffering. It was agonizing. I had never felt so sick. I remembered scarlet fever, a broken arm, a tonsillectomy, the head injury from a head-on car crash, pregnancies and C-sections, asthma attacks, gastritis with nausea, suicidal intervals.

None of them could compare to this.

My legs became terribly sensitive. I couldn't bear the weight of a cover, which was a problem because, as always, I was cold. I shifted my body, trying to find a more comfortable position. Nothing changed the sensation in my legs, but after some minutes I discovered through trial and error that I could rest more easily if my head was elevated somewhere between a forty-five and sixty-degree angle. If I laid very still and closed my eyes, I felt some relief. Otherwise, I was overcome by brain fog or malaise.

I was vaguely aware of falling through the pretense that had been structuring my life as if through a rotting floor and into a dark basement in an abandoned, condemned house. I fell into the shadow that had just become my new reality—into everything I had edited out of my life.

In a way, that's when modernity finally took my body down. In doing so, it created an opening, a way for me to reclaim my true meaning and purpose. There, I surrendered to the end of life as I had known it.

CHAPTER TWO

Engaging the System

—————

I WAS NEVER A TYPICAL DOCTOR.

I had worked to become a doctor from a very early age, but in medical school had watched unattended human suffering pour into the emergency room to be met with life-saving measures that suited a battlefield. As Elizabeth Pisani, author of *The Wisdom of Whores,* put it, we humans treat each other heartlessly until it is too late, and then "come all over compassionate." It was easy to see how healthcare dollars poured into the last year of life. I no longer wanted to save lives that had been given up years or decades earlier. I wanted to identify and mitigate hazards to life so as to help make the last-minute saves unnecessary. I decided to go into preventive medicine, and then into epidemiology and clinical epidemiology research.

I was never even a typical medical researcher.

For example, when I was hired for my first faculty appointment in the Department of Preventive Medicine and Biometrics of the University of Colorado (now the School of Public Health), I heard about a cluster of birth defects and decided to research it. I am the only researcher of my kind that I have known before or since who engaged a real-world problem, rather than one featured in the medical database. I thereby risked losing access to "the big tit"—a sardonic term used by a colleague to refer to the dependable salary and the cozy community that comes of meeting academic expectations. In other words, I would be researching a problem to which I did not already have the answer, which meant that I had no guarantee of solving it. This was not a good career move. One reason that I went ahead was that I was determined to engage the unknown, which is the heart of science.

Furthermore, while most academic doctors rely on the medical database and on standards of care to know what to do, I became one of a small minority of clinical researchers who knows how to identify and interpret its errors. And, as one who took care and cure as objects of study, I had a good idea of what medicine was and wasn't doing well with respect to practice, research, policy, and delivery. I had a big-picture view of its strengths and failings.

Also, I did multidisciplinary work that took me into other areas like medical psychology, diagnostic test evaluation, and environmental health. I joined and went to meetings of the Society for Medical Decision-Making. I knew that in order to succeed as clinicians and researchers, we needed to be clear about the flaws in our reasoning so as to correct them. I felt driven to take heart and to enter the unknown without fear in order to detect unseen hazards and to act accordingly.

I knew that doctors didn't think like scientists and that premodern habits of pattern recognition had been set in stone by centralized management systems. We were still using fancy words like idiopathic and cryptogenic for "I don't know," ostensibly to avoid worrying the patient—but perhaps to bolster ourselves. Chronic disease is, by definition, a failure of prevention as well as treatment, and when typical doctors come up against the unknown and uncertain, they resort unthinkingly to avoidance, denial, and blame. Their fearsome sense of responsibility and the socially-instilled feeling that they should know everything leads most internists to blame themselves, and to feel responsible and ashamed when they don't know what to do—even if no one does. They may then shift the blame to you and become angry, cold, or contemptuous, or shift you to infectious disease or psychiatry. If I hadn't taken a different path, I would have fallen in step.

The context of my first faculty appointment was also unusual.

The community of epidemiologists in Colorado was very small then, and half or so were veterinarians. Those of us who were doctors valued each other and worked collegially and ethically. The woman managing the birth defect investigation welcomed me into her conference room—along with armfuls of regulation books—and said, "Okay. Now let's figure out the right thing to do and then figure out how the regulations justify it." A young philanthropist who heard about the cluster at her salon gave us seed money. The Centers for Disease Control sent out an experienced team of investigators. In medical school, I had taken the course that prepares agents of the Epidemic Intelligence Service (EIS), and was able to join research and medical detecting to engage the unknown—with a freedom unavailable to the EIS, arguably the best group of medical detectives in the world.

In this context, I became one of the minority within a minority of doctors who questions the ideas and methods of clinical research—especially the classification systems and gold standards that we use to define ailments. That is, I sought wisdom and knowledge, as well as information and data, and so used medical databases to serve higher level thinking. I may make a minority of one, being the only one afflicted by one of the emerging epidemics of chronic disease who can—with the help of other unusual doctors—investigate my own case.

While I may be uniquely qualified to do an N-of-1 study of late modern plagues, I was, ironically enough, the worst nightmare of many doctors.

Doctors could not—and still cannot—find my problem in the textbooks or, in any useful way, online. I knew that they could not help me, but I could no longer help myself and felt obliged to participate in the system to the best of my ability. I had seen it work many wonders, as with AIDS, and was unsurprised to find that gay men were some of the few members of the public that grasped what was happening to patients like me—and understood how slowly the system might respond when unprepared and unmotivated.

The night of the crash, I appealed to my husband for help. He was on the faculty of the University of Washington and an internist at the local veteran's hospital. He was board certified in public health and preventive medicine as I was, and was able, in theory, to take what was happening to me as an opportunity to look into an important new epidemic, but he was too busy, and too inclined to take my deterioration as a willful move to make his life more difficult.

He was a man of action, though, and that night, he fed the children and put them to bed. He still had work to do. With me out of commission, three grandparents ailing in various ways, and two young children who were often ill, he was overwhelmed. The stone wall that he had put up around himself to limit his world of responsibilities and his demanding career went to full height that night. He left me to take care of myself and pushed me to do as much for the family as I could.

While he hated it when I talked medicine at home, the night of the crash, and every now and then when I was unable to help myself, he retrieved information for me from online sources. After a brief search, he found the guidelines that the Centers for Disease Control (CDC) had put out in response to the patients flooding into doctors' offices all over the world with new patterns of strange and intractable symptoms. By their criteria, I had "chronic fatigue syndrome (CFS)," for which doctors could do nothing.

I made my way unsteadily upstairs to relieve my symptoms as best I could. I shut the door, turned off the light, and fell into bed. The dark and quiet was a relief. I was keenly sensitive to any kind of stimulation and found it difficult to change position. Lying down and closing my eyes in the dark eased my pain and the discomfort that was like nothing else but could be called a cousin to the flu. I settled into the nightmare of my new life and pondered my diagnostic label. Knowing something about the CDC, I could see behind the magician's curtain. This was big. Really big. The military was seeing it, too, and had labeled it Gulf War Syndrome. It was an epidemic, or, perhaps, a set of epidemics as the CDC criteria implied. A mealy-mouthed diagnosis like fatigue would be their effort to play it down. As they would say in training sessions, the only person who died at the Three Mile Island nuclear emergency was a pregnant woman whose panic led her into a fatal motor crash. Panic kills. The CDC feels responsible for avoiding and mitigating any chance of panic. They were also offering the bare minimum: a provisional case definition. This meant that they had no idea what was going on. We "cases" and our doctors would be on our own.

I knew that my profession was stumped, and that its appeals to other fields to control costs had rendered it helpless. When I had begun my training in the 70's, doctors had just started to "treat the chart." This put the virtual patient before the real patient, and supported a growing bureaucracy of third-party players: economists, lawyers, and managers who imagined they had it all under control. They exerted this control with the advent of information systems that excluded grey areas and eventually precluded thought and problem-solving. No patient could avoid this interference. I had to accept it. Were I not entered into the system as a diagnostic label, my case would not exist from the point of view of society. I would not qualify for any kind of support from the late modern system of medical care. I would disappear into the gap between reality and virtual reality.

So, the next morning, after dropping the kids at school and at daycare, and being obliged to stop at the side of the road for an episode of the dry heaves, I called the local clinic. I thought that because I lived in a small town, and my children and mother went to that clinic, they might see me in the urgent care area. But the phone number led to a robotic scheduler at the affiliated Virginia Mason Hospital in Seattle, and, as I was not in their system, the earliest appointment they would offer was three months away. I considered showing up at urgent care, but having no way of telling how long I might have to wait or how much it would set me back, I decided against it. I had to save what little energy I had for the kids. I once again appealed to my husband. He was well connected and found a top internist at an elite city clinic who would, as a personal favor to him, see me the following week.

That would give me time to prepare; my main problem was that I had every symptom in the book, which was not very specific and would trigger suspicion. People try to get medical care for all kinds of strange reasons. In my training, I had encountered fake stories concocted by criminals who wanted to get into the hospital to evade custody, people who ran out of money for food, family members who were trying to get rid of someone they didn't like or couldn't handle, and child-like adults who wanted to please by saying yes to everything. Admitting that I had a universally positive review of systems, as we call the checklist at the end of the full history and physical, would trigger suspicion. Scapegoating had already become a problem for me. Most doctors were contemptuous of patients with my condition. We were seen as head cases or malingerers.

On the day of my appointment, I made my way in our new car via the ferry to the Capitol Hill neighborhood where we had lived when we first moved to Seattle from Chicago in 1982. The hospital parking garage was new, and so space efficient that I dented the new car. My coordination wasn't what it had been. I felt like I was eighty years old, and perhaps was beginning to drive that way. This was characteristic: I had many problems that fell within the range of "normal" for many patients but were way outside my own normal. I took the elevator up, found my doctor's lobby, and was ushered into the examining room. Even before the doctor entered I knew he would be competent and personable. Seattle was lousy with doctors; to join a strong practice like this, he had to have impeccable credentials and a manageable ego.

And indeed, he came in precisely on time, greeted me kindly, and took a seat. He was of medium height, with dark hair and beard, and in the prime of life. Alert but not edgy, confident but not arrogant, plain-spoken but technically savvy, he positioned the familiarity of his manner between professional courtesy—impossible in Seattle, where so many patients were doctors—and pure professionalism. I relaxed and told him my story in a way that I hoped had a chance of making enough medical sense that he might be able to help me.

I began, tongue in cheek, like a third-year medical student presenting my case, "The patient was perfectly well until..."

I told him that I had begun having problems toward the end of my first pregnancy in Denver. I had stopped being able to walk to work, not because of any problems with mobility or a fear of falling on ice, but because I couldn't hold my bowels. This continued after delivery and worsened over time. I had been a vegetarian for years, and enjoyed spicy foods, but no matter how conservatively I ate, I was subject to explosive watery diarrhea, bloating, nausea, and food intolerances, beginning with corn on the cob. I had gone to a gastroenterologist who gave me medication to suppress my symptoms. Whatever the underlying problem might be, the medication didn't stop it. It did relieve some symptoms at the cost of making it impossible for me to tell what else might make me better or worse, information I could have used to detect the cause.

As time went on, I developed the butterfly rash of lupus, plus itchy bumps on my hands and nape. I developed depression, for which I took an SSRI (sertraline) that also suppressed my symptoms. With a concerted effort, I was able to taper and then discontinue all those meds, which enabled me to follow the natural history of my illness.

I had also developed asthma, which was difficult to detect because my only symptom was loss of exercise tolerance while walking in nature—for years I had thought I was only losing fitness due to debility from my chronic condition.

More recently, I had developed neurological symptoms. In addition to the brain fog that seemed to reflect problems of the central nervous system, I had peripheral nerve pain, problems with balance, and the pill-rolling tremor of Parkinson's. This was on top of a lifelong "glass" or "fine" tremor. Most of all, I had hard-to-pinpoint autonomic nervous system symptoms, including slow and incomplete urination, lid lag, difficulty swallowing, and difficulty equilibrating after standing.

I also had a variety of other problems such as recurrent vaginal yeast, the treatment of which seemed to make me feel worse; ulcers and blood blisters in my mouth; and headaches, sore throats, and insomnia.

The doctor examined me, ordered lab tests, and asked me to return the following week.

After being ushered into his examining room for the second time, he tapped lightly on the door and walked in, hand out. He shook my hand and we said hellos. He took a seat at his desk and looked at my lab results.

He began to stroke his chin. As he riffled through my chart, he began to frown. I knew from professional experience what he was doing: He was trying to find patterns among and within the symptoms, signs, and lab results so that he could come up with a list of tentative diagnoses to rule out—or rule in, and possibly treat. He was trying to match my illness to known patterns he had studied and memorized in medical school or in the course of continuing education. He was excluding "The Known."

I sat there, patiently waiting for him to finish reading.

When he had finished, he looked up at me. "You have the tremor that you've had all your life, and you have a high bilirubin, low white count, and high steroid levels, but you've had those before."

I said as bravely as I could, "It's okay. I couldn't figure it out either."

He said, "Your lab tests show that you're fine. All you have is the fatigue."

"Fatigue? What fatigue? I'm sick, with an unknown and mysterious problem."

"You meet the criteria for chronic fatigue syndrome."

"Yes. I meet the provisional case definition."

There was a ponderous silence. He, like my husband before him, looked stricken. "I'm sorry. There's nothing I can do."

"Can we try some kind of investigation, or experimental treatment?"

He looked ashamed. "I'm sorry, but there's no treatment."

I was taken aback. He was firing me. That would happen time and time again with internists. There would be no bearing witness to my experience, no counseling, no trying anything. At least this one was kind. That would prove to be unusual. I understood the reasons, but I didn't like it that failure and helplessness were so integral to state-of-the-art care. It wasn't good enough and we all knew it.

"Thank you for your time," I said.

He nodded grimly as I walked out.

At least now I was in the system as a CFS patient, which made me eligible to participate in a federally-funded research study on the disease. I was very fortunate to live in Seattle because it was the site of one of only two centers for the study of "chronic fatigue" in existence at the time. And the principal investigator—I'll call her Dr. D—was one of the very few in the country who had been willing to legitimize the diagnosis by taking it as a subject of study.

Dr. D, a rarity in a division of internists that was still, for the most part, a boy's club, was a sharp, savvy, pragmatic activist who could see the problem of CFS through more than one frame of reference. She knew that the new epidemics were impacting women's health, and was willing and able to stand up and do something about it. That meant organizing—in the best tradition of academics—a proposal that would get funded and still give her a chance to do some good.

In the profession, chronic fatigue syndrome had taken the place of hysteria and neurasthenia, stigmatizing labels that blamed women for their illnesses and let doctors off the hook. Because of this, she would face ingrained sexism and risk contempt for appearing to gratify head cases and malingerers with a serious response that they didn't deserve. It was a tough political tack to take. She would have to please everyone who needed pleasing to get the study done.

Fortunately she was equal to the task, and she had some support at the National Institutes of Health (NIH), where the staff recognized their duty to respond to the needs of the new wave of patients.

I was eager to support her work, and made an appointment

to see her as soon as possible. Weeks later, arriving for my intake visit, I met: Dr. D; a psychologist colleague who researched insomnia; and a male radiologist who had been among the first cases and had volunteered to do a research project of his own. I also met her care team and took advantage of resources that other patients had left for their peers on the shelves in the waiting area.

I received some very good practical advice when the occupational therapist told me it was possible to rest *too much*. When you feel as bad as a CFS sufferer feels, your instinct is to take a lot of breaks. You think "My body needs to rest. If I lie down, I'll feel better." But this could spawn a downward spiral into debility. My background was preventive medicine, so I knew that exercise was necessary as well as a panacea. I was already walking every day I could, but this conversation helped me to figure out a better balance between rest and activity. The doctor also advised against applying for disability insurance: The university offered a poor policy for its faculty, and going through the hoops they had set up to create a "proof of illness" was a kind of torture that was best to avoid if at all possible.

After I had spent one hour filling out personality profiles and other psychological questionnaires, I asked the insomnia investigator, "Aren't you going to ask anything about reproductive history? Word has it that onset is usually post-partum. Mine was. And I have Gilbert's syndrome, a heritable condition with chronic high bilirubin. Plus, I had a head injury and worked in a sick building where other women got fibromyalgia, MS, and other illnesses."

He looked embarrassed. "We don't have the funding."

My jaw dropped. I knew that it would have cost next to

nothing to add a few questions about the physical body.

But after I saw Doctor D, she said, "Oh! You have a history of head injury," referring to the car crash that had rendered me unconscious for a few hours. "You're not eligible for the study."

I suspected that she was being kind by giving me an excuse to lift my stigma, but I was having none of it. I wanted to know the real cause, and when I asked more questions she explained, "This isn't a causal study. We don't know where the cases come from and can't get a control group." I knew the methodological issues as well as my own name. I also knew that a doable study was the only way to begin, and to justify doing a better one. It soon came out that this was a follow-up study with a psychiatric hypothesis: Patients who weren't better in a year were expected to have begun with a bad attitude that fit one or more diagnostic labels in psychology or psychiatry. I don't know whether I was more disappointed to be excluded or to have my time wasted by a study with such an agenda.

But I went back for a few visits, and Doctor D was able to show cerebellar abnormalities on physical exam in me and in many other patients, and to find enough twins to produce data suggestive of a genetic predisposition to CFS—hard findings that doctors could get their minds around. I tried to look enthused, but I had seen many investigators go after genes and end up finding none—or too many to comprehend. And I knew the epidemics that were arising and spreading so fast couldn't be explained by genes. From my point of view, the attitude of the system was so bad that it was crippling itself.

But I was better off than I had been. Through the clinic, I got onto a CDC email list that was supporting a dialogue between doctor-patients and doctors. Much of the continuing conversation consisted of doctors who wanted the CDC to help their isolated communities, or who were despairing because they had nothing to offer their endlessly hopeful patients. But as I couldn't help the isolated docs—some from as far away as New Zealand—and didn't want to get entangled in doctors' complaints, I gave it up. I didn't want to spend my time caring for the system that was not caring for me.

~

In so many ways, medical systems have been the proudest achievement of the late modern era: Emergency medicine services; monitoring and control of dangerous communicable diseases; and Nixon's war on heart disease, cancer, and stroke are among the efforts that have saved countless lives. But the systems that respond so adroitly to selected metrics, and consequently create the desired data, are unresponsive to rapidly changing biological realities and model helpless fatalism. One prominent physician told me that the system would work in thirty years, and that I should wait. He seemed oblivious to the fact that I had been in pain for years; that I would probably be gone long before then; and that the system was already failing. It was inhumane, unaffordable, and spectacularly unsuccessful in coping with the new plagues.

And so, even though my brain was off-line, I could do better on my own. First, I could try. Second, I could get ambitious. I could drop the idea the chronic illness had no causes and could go for preventive cure.

I kept thinking back to the night of my crash for encouragement. I realized that I was a researcher dedicated to uncovering the causes of a disease, and a medical detective who knew what to do. It dawned on me as I lay there alone in the darkness that first night that I was getting exactly what I had asked for: a chance to explore a new and unknown plague.

CHAPTER THREE

Reclaiming the Intangible

———

FOR THE FIRST COUPLE OF WEEKS, I spent the daylight hours walking and laying in bed as much as possible, watching television until I couldn't stomach it, and then lying with my laptop on my hips, writing. My father had taught me to write in primary school, when he at times obliged me to stay at my desk. Later I had stopped because I felt I had nothing to write about.

Now I had plenty. Like most doctors, I had not taken time to process all that I had gone through. The unexamined backlog of experience—especially my college years on the South Side of Chicago—rose like a living nightmare. I began to write it all out, which kept me from having an existential crisis—or, rather, gave my processing a constructive and cathartic outlet. Writing also helped me apply my mind and emotions to a task that I could do with brain fog, because I had nothing at stake and could do it again and again as the state of my nervous system allowed.

When the family was home, I did my best to keep up with my responsibilities. I would drag myself out of bed in the morning after a painful, relatively sleepless night, get the kids ready, and drive them to school and daycare. Then I would do what needed to be done to hand off my research project, such as make phone calls and send emails to a colleague in the East who was kind enough to finish the analysis and write up the results with the top-notch staff who had worked on the study. Then I would rest, and on good days make dinner for my family and clean up afterward.

But doing laundry was my *tour de force*. That's how far my life had shrunk. I would load the dirty clothes into the washer. I would load the wet, clean clothes into the dryer. I would take the dry clothes out, fold them, and put them away. No matter how bad things got, I at least did this—no matter how much it hurt. To do less would be to admit I was finished, to say that I was giving up on life. And sadly, I was close to doing so.

Physically, I was in what I came to see as a state worse than death. There was no moment of the day that I was not aware of—and defined by—pain, nausea, and distress. I tried to conceal it from others, but could not conceal it from my own awareness. Because of this, I made a pact with myself: If after one year, I did not have some time in the day when I could disregard my symptoms, I would commit suicide. In the meantime, I would do everything I possibly could do to feel better.

As my life stabilized into this new routine, I began to explore self-healing. After reading *Spontaneous Healing* by Dr. Andrew Weil, I set aside time every day to do a visualization guided by audio recordings by Belleruth Naparstek, or Joan Borysenko.

Although in the beginning these visualizations only eased my pain and suffering while I was doing them, and for short intervals after, as time passed the benefit lasted longer and would return whenever I thought about the visualization. I soon realized that visualization was conditioning my body and being, and the conditioning that relieved suffering (which Buddhists call "the pain of the pain") was progressing more quickly than the conditioning that was relieving the pain itself. I recognized that if my healing journey became a spiritual one. I would be able to make better progress, eventually becoming able to heal the intangible body, and through it, my immune system. If my illness was the result of an infectious agent of some kind, the healing might even effect a cure. I also learned a little about Buddhism, and recognized this potential for self-care and cure as the self-care of the Buddha, who was sometimes called "the supreme physician."

I gradually recognized that writing was calling me back to unresolved trauma and distress that were pulling me down like sandbags, and understood that in order to stay afloat, I would have to cast them off. These weights included the loss of the work for which I had striven my whole life; stories of shame, guilt, fear, and despair that my inner doctor was all too happy to punish me for; and loss of almost all of the social connections I had not already given up. I felt isolated and abandoned, and worst of all, my profession had let me down in every possible way. It was hell.

Fortunately, I had not lost all. I had my family. My mother supported me emotionally. My husband's status and income protected me from poverty and from scapegoating by the medical system. Our children warmed our hearts. Two neighboring families and a handful of long-time friends also continued to include me in their lives.

With the support that I had, and the support of the cultures I was now learning about, I was able to pursue intangible healing through ancient traditions that were at one time the sole source of care and cure, and which were useful enough to be kept alive into our own time. I had soon learned many practices from a variety of traditions and had added those that were most effective to my repertory of self-help skills.

 Along the way, I discovered meditation and prayer classes filled with seekers who had been failed by late-modern doctors and clergy, and who were exploring states of wonder and ways of knowing rejected by moderns. By the end of the first year, I was in a good enough state to ignore my illness most mornings. I was learning as much about faith, practice, and theology as I had ever learned about anything, other than biomedicine, and was thrilled with the new vistas it opened. I was sure that the way to care and cure would be discovered through aspects of the human experience that doctors and researchers were ignoring, and I immersed myself in them. Ultimately, these aspects formed the patterns that shaped my emerging process of discovery—much as Arianism and alchemy had formed the patterns that enabled Newton to transform old ways of seeing into new ones.

Over the following years, while fellow patients were prescribed cognitive behavioral theory, I found myself spending time with hundreds of people who were engaged in personal transformation from the inside out. This included keepers of ancient paths to rebirth in illness, and those who were forming their own paths with a community. Emulating Maimonides, I scoured every tradition I could find for items that I could stow in an expanding tool bag for realizing care and cure. While my former colleagues focused on one hot molecule after another, ignoring the other million that might matter more than the ones filling their awareness, I was pursuing and integrating a cultural, global, and historic search for effective practices for self-care and treatments for self-cure.

The following is a look at a few key moments of discovery in this unexpectedly—to me—fruitful phase of my case study.

⁓

Late on a Friday afternoon in cool, cloudy weather, I was with a carload of people heading west toward Harmony House, a retreat center on the Hood Canal. Dedicated to people recovering from cancer, in the low season this center also offered retreats to people with other illnesses to help make ends meet. We would be participating in a weekend silent retreat with exchange of Reiki, which was easy to learn and ideal for people who wanted to use touch therapy to help a sick or dying family member feel better. While this retreat was intended for bodyworkers of various kinds, and I was a neophyte, I had heard that there were spaces left and had been allowed to tag along.

As it got dark, the four of us who were carpooling together shared personal stories, and I realized that while none of us had cancer, we each had reasons to seek healing. One woman was a dancer whose passion for ballet had ended in her teens with severe arthritis. Another was a DES daughter—that is, her mother had taken diethylstilbestrol during pregnancy— who struggled with reproductive health issues. We would find out that another retreatant had come out as gay and suffered crushing rejection. One had multiple sclerosis. One had an ankle injury, another had back pain. A few simply wanted to practice as much as possible.

After arriving and unpacking in our rooms, we shared a nourishing, chatty dinner. As we gathered in the library a bit later, all in good spirits, our group felt generally relaxed and relieved, and with eyes sparkling in the low light we played a few games, like angel cards, to edge us all gently into a contemplative state. Following this, the retreat leader explained the weekend schedule: During the day, we would meet in the yurts near the house and trade Reiki for several-hour intervals. Each time, we were to choose someone we hadn't treated yet, with both people giving and receiving. When we were not doing Reiki or eating meals, we were to enjoy the outdoor gardens and seashell labyrinth, or walk farther afield, perhaps to the waterfront park down the road. From the end of this meeting until late Sunday afternoon, when we would gather again, we would not speak, read, or otherwise use language or engage others. We were to let our minds go quiet.

I had been to other silent retreats and would go to many more, but this was unique for the depth of silence we could obtain. In clergy-run retreats, there were usually teaching sessions, readings, private or group counseling, or discussion. These continually activated the language center of the brain that governs expressive and receptive speech. At this retreat, we would rest the language center and allow the silence to deepen progressively.

I had read and heard of the value of inner silence, but words could not convey the taste of it, nor give a glimpse of the world in which some sages abide. There is peace in the absence of language, and especially in the absence of the thousands of repetitive or useless habits that may have formed in the mind in the past. These may have been maladaptive at their beginning or have long since become obsolete; in that way, the mind can be like an attic filled with forgotten and broken items all covered with cobwebs, silverfish, mold, and rat remains. This much may be easy to imagine, and a pleasure to be rid of for any length of time.

What I couldn't imagine, and in fact could barely apprehend, was the recognition of brain activity that had been masked by my prima-donna-like language center. Here was an uninterrupted wealth of inner life beyond any of the five senses as well as the cognitive, the emotional, and the kinesthetic. I encountered raw being, the puniness of the modern "structuring" of raw experience, and the untapped possibilities of existence. I recognized that humans hold endless untapped possibilities of joy, connection, perception, and direct experience that we might yet comprehend and put to good use.

Toward the end of the silent period, as I walked along the main road to the park and passed some strangers who greeted me in a friendly way, I opened my mouth to reply—but nothing came out. It took what seemed a very long time to produce a delayed hello. That was the end of the deep silence, and by the time we retreatants met for the last time, my language center—Broca's area of the left cerebral cortex, at least—was active again, and the rest of my mind was back in shadow. But I now knew what resided within, and the potential of inner silence for the development of experiential learning.

$$\sim$$

Asian classical civilizations—especially in India—had developed a treasure house of traditions enabling adepts to intervene in the flesh. In particular the tantric practices that originated in India enable the individual to accelerate becoming and to alter doing. For example, *tonglen* can transform trauma into joy, and *tummo* enables monks to dress lightly in arctic weather. Most Westerners imagine that such intangible practices are ineffective—except, perhaps, when they encounter an advanced martial artist like Bruce Lee who uses energetics interpersonally. In fact, you can learn to use the focus of your awareness to discover the subtle inner structures of the energy body and harness them for healing. You can change your life—if you have the patient humility to seek out the right teacher and to collect the skills that you need, and if illness has not disabled your focus or depleted your energy.

Most such traditions have, until very recently, been locked up by vows of secrecy. As East meets West, some have been gradually released, such as the *chenrezig* visualization and embodiment practice that the fourteenth Dalai Lama made available to all. As martial arts courses reveal, some practices can be dangerous and have traditionally been conveyed only to students who have mastered their prerequisites. Some time ago, however, a master practitioner, Mantak Chia, put all of his Daoist teachings into books that have been translated into English.

At one local store sponsored by an *ashram,* I asked for advice and was taken to a shelf filled with Chia's books. A keeper of the Thai Royal tradition of esoteric work, he offered practices for many purposes such as fertility, spiritual expression, and healing. All I knew at the time was that his methods looked precise, felt authentic, promised healing, and were new to me. I had had good results with Qi Gong, but this was my first attempt to use my mind to alter my energy body, and I was jumping in at the deep end. All I had were some useful skills, a knowledge of anatomy, and plenty of time to practice. Fortunately for me, that was enough.

I soon discovered that my energy body seemed to be fragmented and diffuse, and its core weak. It turned out that I could use the easiest practice to strengthen the central channel that runs along the front of the spine, and the energy centers along it, such as the navel center. I had heard the phrase "navel gazing," and had used those words dismissively without knowing their esoteric origins. After wincing to think of my ignorance, I applied this practice to do what my body no longer did automatically: bring my energy to the center where it could strengthen my flesh and being.

Eventually, I found that I could circulate energy in through my eyes and ears and down to my navel center and pelvis; I could also bring my awareness into contact with my gut, which had gradually become an insensate void. And while I saw how this practice could be used for harm—for me it was a kind of respite care that I was able to offer my ailing body.

I later consulted Harrison Moretz, a local adept who had told me not to return to his Qi Gong class because circulating energy was—at that time—interfering with the health of my energy body. When I mentioned Chia, he became upset and told me a cautionary tale about an adept he knew who had tried the celibacy practice and lost his erection for many more weeks than expected. I wondered why a man might use it if he expected it to fail, but I took his point: energy work is not to be undertaken lightly.

I came to think of many kinds of inner work as self-patterning or emerging embodied psychology. Chia's approach made use of the energy body and required long, intensive practice that develops many skills, such as relaxation, advanced body mindfulness, and creation of an intense pinpoint focus of concentration. When students become able to create a strong pea-sized focus, they can learn to move it anywhere in the body at will. Eventually they can move it through the channels of the energy body and locate energy nexi such as the heart chakras. This is far more difficult than taking a pill. Also, it is not without risk, and it removes the intangible benefits offered by a human carer. For someone with chronic illness who spends only a tiny percentage of time in care, however, this is well worth attempting with prudence and with whatever useful support is available (for more, see *The Chronic Illness Owner's Manual.*)

～

For intellectual self-patterning, I turned to Judaism. In college, I had noticed that my closest intellectual friends were Jewish, and my most accomplished professors had left Europe before or during the Holocaust, now called the *Shoah*. One day a student in theoretical physics confessed to me that he couldn't think of a single great scientist or philosopher who wasn't Jewish. When I mentioned Newton he seemed greatly relieved. I understood his perspective, but it wasn't until I became involved with the multifaith community in Seattle, and much later read *The Burnt Book* by Marc-Alain Ouaknin that I discovered the esoteric religious practices that seem to have patterned so many Jewish thinkers—including the secular Jewish Nobel Prize winners of last century.

Serendipitously, as part of exploring the esoteric healing practices of world traditions, I began to attend retreats organized by The Interfaith Amigos, one of whom is Rabbi Ted

Falcon, author of *A Journey of Awakening*. This book features an annual practice of embodying the tree of life in a way strongly influence by Maimonides, who integrated medicine and Judaism in the middle ages, and whose teachings are still used. To oversimplify, it is a way of locating Godly—that is, inherent—ethics and virtues in the body and balancing them, and also of inviting heavenly—that is, uplifting—wisdom to manifest on Earth. This can be used as self-patterning for discovery and problem-solving.

Another method I encountered may have patterned the likes of Tversky and Kahneman, whose work on expert judgment makes it possible to detect and remedy systematic cognitive errors: the tradition of open-ended, non-ideological dialogue that avoids consensus—especially the premature consensus arising when investigators think too much alike. When thinking and engaging in non-ideological, non-consensus dialogue, it is the truth that wins rather than a person—so far as a seeker or a pair of seekers can discover the truth.

When combined with compassionate listening, the dialogue can become contemplative and sacred, and compatible with care as well as cure. Sacred contemplative dialogue is less destructive to ideas than is the ritual combat of debate. It can even be used for peacemaking, and is therefore conducive to shared as well as individual problem-solving. Retreating from the brink of extinction will require a letting-go of heated conflict combined with discovery of old and new tools of every kind that engage all aspects of body and being. Evolving these tools may catalyze change fast enough and well enough to avert the Sixth Extinction.

$\sim$

And so, by pursuing the ultimate self-help of personal transformation from the inside out, I was able to reach into the Jungian shadow side of modernity (i.e. that which we ignore) and to learn to appreciate and care for the whole of my body. Rather than try to turn back the clock, I turned to deep time, gathered the discoveries of the ancestors, and put the past century into perspective.

Eventually, I realized that the pattern that I was following as I worked had come from several sources. I could hold a working question in my awareness (Gurdjieff); allow my energy to flow down from above my head through apprehension, comprehension, and what I came to call perceptions (Tantra and Judaism); and direct my course toward a vision (derived from Gurdjieff). This became my theosophical path, and supported me in discovery. In this I was following in the footsteps of quasi-esotericists such as Newton and Einstein, who were patterned by philosophy and theology. Like those scientists and esotericists who hold all of creation as sacred and view it with wonder, I abided in a state that invites scientific revelation.

CHAPTER FOUR

Searching the Globe

―――――

M Y OBJECT WAS TO LEAVE NO STONE UNTURNED in search for the treatments that worked. Fortunately, this came naturally as I had always been a practical idealist. For one thing, my mother was from Sweden and was characteristically well grounded in the nitty-gritty realities of everyday life. For another, though I had no religious or spiritual affiliation, I was strongly influenced by secular Jewish friends who had taken the universe as their Torah, and who lived the principle of world healing called *tikkun olam*, an effort intensified by the Holocaust, now called the Shoah. I had been born into a related situation in that my father—thirteen generations after his Puritan ancestors had brought dissent to this shore—had been a prisoner of war for three years in Nazi Germany. As a child, I couldn't help ease his post-traumatic stress disorder, but my efforts to do so set a pattern of trying to fix the unfixable, to cure what I could feel but couldn't understand.

As with intangible forms of self-help, tangible ones from all cultures were spreading rapidly as modern medicine failed to respond to "The New." I was therefore able to consult practitioners from all over the globe without leaving town. Many used paradigms that had begun in antiquity during the Axial Age, that is the time of the Sramana, Buddha, Prophets, and

Lao Tzu, the first known do-it-yourself movement that spread through the grassroots around the globe. In this search, I had help from medical doctors who had been exploring what some call alternative, complementary, or integrative medicine. Below follow a few key examples of what I encountered here in the states—and abroad—during this continuing exploration.

∾

Even before I got in to see a medical doctor, I called Bastyr University and made an appointment to see a practitioner of Asian medicine. At the time, Bastyr had just become one of two federally-funded "alternative" medical schools in the country, and was incorporating faculty from the Northwest Institute of Oriental Medicine, a school of Naturopathy, and instructors who taught the basic sciences. Still small, its clinic was located above a restaurant in the Wallingford neighborhood of Seattle, with its own pharmacy downstairs from the clinic.

When I was taken into a patient room, two students came in to see me. One was a former Air Force medic, the other a Thai man who had studied conventional Western medicine in China and was now studying traditional Chinese medicine at Bastyr. Together they had extensive experience of the world. Upon meeting them, I thought "what an interesting cultural crossover!" And although I didn't realize it then, this same kind of boundary crossing, which went way beyond my previous multidisciplinary work, would become a big part of my quest for care and cure.

As the students took my detailed history, I noticed how different their approach was to Western medical practice. While they did ask many questions about my prior health conditions, their primary focus was on my *now*. They took my pulses. They looked at my tongue. They wanted to know what I was feeling. I gradually began to understand that they would treat my state of being directly, and in that way I would be a different patient every time I had an appointment. It wasn't until later that I understood it as a hybrid of Western and Eastern medicine that modeled hands-on care as a way of relieving suffering by enhancing a patient's well-being.

After the history and examination, they went away and analyzed my case. They came back and told me I had a chi deficiency of the spleen, and because my sexual function was still okay, they said my energy should get better. But *that* was their diagnosis—chi deficiency of the spleen. I had never heard anything like it.

Then Dr. Cao came in. He was the attending faculty member and had practiced Oriental Medicine in Beijing for thirty years before coming to the states. He was very kind, and very concerned. He said, "We don't know what you have. But we're going to try to help you."

I relaxed. They did not withdraw, condescend, or punish. I didn't have a shameful condition. I nearly burst into tears.

They were smart. They were not afraid of the unknown. And they were willing to try to help me. The latter two qualities were a far cry from what I met with in the late-modern, high tech, Western medical system.

That visit to Bastyr was wonderful. It was nurturing, validating, inspiring, *and* encouraging. And I could continue treatments as long as I chose.

During that visit I had my first-ever treatment with acupuncture, supervised by a doctor who had learned, practiced, and taught Oriental medicine at its source. I felt my good fortune. The treatment used Japanese needles, and took twenty minutes. It is hard to describe how it felt. The needle sticks were nothing compared to those of modern allopathic medical needles, and I could feel a change that was subtle and intangible. Not better or worse; just different.

Later that day I was very relaxed. That night I slept soundly. Over the next few days, I felt "knocked out." And then I began to feel better. Over the next few months, my treatments seemed to shift my state of being away from adrenal overload.

~

When I talked to my project manager at the National Institutes of Health, Dr. Locke, it turned out that he was working on CFS in children, and that his roots traced back to a small village in China. I thought that he might express interest in Asian medicine, but when I told him that acupuncture helped, he said, "Oh, placebo effect, I suppose."

My reply? "Well, I hope so! I need all the placebo I can get!"

Scientists think of placebo in a very magical way, and they don't like it. The word itself was invented when researchers discovered that subjects could get better when they thought they were getting a drug they believed in, even if they had only received a sugar pill. That is, scientists were dismayed to find that what test subjects expected changed test outcomes. They did their best to get rid of this uncontrollable factor—which may have been deep Pavlovian conditioning, good will, or something else—and called it the placebo effect.

Dr. Locke sighed, and told me that the NIH was beginning to see the value of harnessing the placebo effect and to fund research on the topic. And as I began to do my own work with this, I took my first step toward owning my own placebo, which moved me closer to turning my life into a case study that included continual interventions or self-care and that would eventually extend to self-cure.

～

Another example of my search for tangible treatments occurred several years later, when I splurged and spent money on care and decided to spend a week at an elite spa in Arizona during the hot season, when guest packages were on sale. I flew to Tucson and took the dedicated shuttle to what looked like a fancy resort in the shadow of a minor, shower-prone mountain. It reminded me a bit of Disneyland in that there were "backstage" areas for staff and a carefully landscaped campus—in this case still surrounded by the natural world.

The spa was luxurious. There was an equine facility with an obstacle course, and other features dedicated to corporate retreats. There was a full-service spa with the latest in wraps, facials, and mud baths for visitors from Los Angeles. And there was a place where people with chronic illness could come to learn self-care. After receiving a reading via intuitive Reiki, I was given a personalized curriculum that included a world of treatments and practices. I was in heaven.

I tried a Daoist dynamic meditation, Qi Gong, and Daoist teachings; an Ayurvedic assessment for type of constitution and diet, as well as meditation and yoga; a chiropractic craniosacral massage; talk therapy; a spa bath; a delicious and nutritious menu of healthy gourmet food; walks on trails; and a shamanic rite. I also had a luxury cabin where I could go whenever I wanted to sleep, nap, watch teaching videos, or read inspirational literature. It was like a low-stress sampler of world medical traditions. They were all wonderful, though some were also harrowing and cathartic. I didn't want to leave.

But when I did leave, I was able to continue my search through global traditions in Seattle, where there were dedicated practitioners keeping the best of the human past alive and evolving. For the first decade, I did a self-study course in the global history of medicine wherever I went.

I soon discovered, though, that the providers of various modalities of care and cure were like the blind men and the elephant: They saw only one aspect of the body and thought the rest an extension of it. Even in the most advanced integrative medicine clinics, various practitioners were unable to communicate with one another. It was as if each were treating a different species. And so, like other patients, I had to make sense of it all myself.

~

A decade on, I consulted a family practitioner who practiced with a naturopath. The doctor was compassionate, open-minded, experimental, and constantly afraid of having his license pulled for practicing in an unconventional way—as has happened to other like-minded doctors who begin to think and act in ways out of step with the system.

Pretty soon I was spending up to four hundred dollars a month on visits, tests, and interventions, and above all on supplements. I even received an IV injection of glutathione that overrode all my symptoms for one hour. And because my doctor's partner had the same condition and was continually experimenting on herself, she was able to share what she had tried and felt worked. This was the perfect medical practice for me, and I was happy to sign on, take the risk, and go along for the ride.

Everything seemed to help a little bit—and one thing helped a lot: Almost right away the doctor prescribed a temporary liquid diet for bowel rest. Then, over time, he diagnosed leaky bowel, and continued to adjust my treatment. Leaky bowel was the one instance in which doctors who wanted to get naturopaths to do their work were richly rewarded: A new clinical condition was recognized, defined, and effectively treated by going around the conventional medical system. Leaky bowel is common, and its treatment is big business.

With an elimination diet and a course of an over-the-counter liquid diet powder, my rash cleared; my bloating, nausea, mouth sores, gingivitis, and other digestive symptoms eased; and I felt relief. My health and well-being really took a step up. After the liquid diet, however, the symptoms would gradually begin again, and I found that when I used a powder that included an immune suppressant, I would get better faster *and* get sicker faster. There was inflammation in my gut, and the treatment was more like a Band-Aid than a cure. Something was causing my gut—and my lungs—to be inflamed, and it wasn't the foods that an allergist had eliminated from my diet. It was something else that I couldn't imagine.

Eventually, this experimental practice focused only on chronic Lyme disease. I took many courses of high-dose antibiotics, which eased some symptoms and caused others. My microbiome was hard hit, with the probiotic supplements that I was taking to offset it only adding to my problems. And I was still sick.

I began to doubt the methods and conclusions behind the Lyme diagnosis. My doctor, who had a tendency to take everything as confirming his hypothesis, was not trained in clinical or public health epidemiology. And neither practitioner grasped the basic concepts of the causal web, diagnostic test evaluation, or systematic treatment evaluation. The diagnosis and treatment seemed to me to be off-target and strongly influenced by the groupthink and wishful thinking of doctors who were trying to compensate for the system. I soon decided to move on.

～

I started thinking about medical history, cultures, and paradigms, how cultures solve or don't solve medical problems, and what happens to them as a result. I soon realized that every surviving culture throughout the history of humankind has used a unique combination of tangible and intangible care in solving its health problems. I also came to understand that if a culture is unable to solve its problems of body and being, it is likely to cease to exist.

The modern focus on tangible structure—which began with the resurrection of autopsies in the early modern era, increasing until it became counterproductive—was an outlier in the history of the species. And it has not become a part of the necessary past; it is a swing of the pendulum that has allowed us to discover the limits of focusing exclusively on the flesh. The separation of the tangible and intangible aspects of the nervous system that followed Drs. Charcot, Babinsky, Freud, and James is untenable. My case study—as I came to view my search for cure—would have to be put into the context of the big picture of place and time.

I began to recognize the emerging epidemics that included my case as markers of the end of post-post modernism and, I now understood, the start of a new era. It signaled an epochal change like those attributed to Hippocrates, Galen, Avicenna, Maimomides, Vesalius, and to the doctors of the Scottish Enlightenment. And, as before, this was precipitated by illnesses—like the bubonic plague that gave birth to the modern era—along with other problems that would end the era. This meant that the frames and constructs of the new era would provide the point of view from which to see the limitations of the old. Fortunately, this new worldview—which some call the emerging paradigm—was already coming into being all around the globe, especially in permaculture, agriculture, architecture, and localism, all of which were blossoming in Seattle along with the final expressions of modernity that were bridging the gap—the first experiments in information technology among them.

While so-called alternative or integrative medical practices were flourishing locally, the frames and constructs that underpinned them were limited by paradigm capture of one kind or another. Many were "turning back the clock" and relying on premodern paradigms; others were reviving chiropractic and homeopathic paradigms from the modern era; and still others were anchored on the gold standard of anatomy revealed by less invasive and more detailed new technologies analogous to X-ray fluoroscopy but assumed to be harmless, such as MRI.

Eerily, while my illness had seemed to burn out the "data-processing" aspect of my nervous system, and so made it impossible for me to remain in the modern workplace, it had seemed to preserve—perhaps even augment—the higher order functions that educators refer to as information, knowledge, and wisdom. I also had a storehouse of life experience and was—with intangible healing—able to form new memories and to read selected emotionally intelligent books. So I had time on my hands and the tools I needed to do the conceptual work that would create new frames and constructs. I could become what I thought of as a "real" professor—unpaid, and unbound by the role of employee, with the potential to transform suffering into solutions that mattered.

So I began to construct a framework—an emerging medical paradigm—that could support new diagnoses and treatments that were at once preventive and curative. This paradigm began with a new view of the body. With respect to the global history of medicine, this view was integrative, combining the wisdom of India with respect to the intangible body (the five aspects of ancient times plus the energy body of the classical period); the modern allopathic understanding of the flesh on the clinical human scale (with a renewed focus on organ systems); and interbeing as proposed by Thich Nhat Hanh and modeled by ecologists. This construct allowed me to incorporate those old human forms of care and cure that I encountered.

By adding the construct of nested bodies, I was also able to take advantage of the care and cure offered freely by the beleaguered but still generous body of life. This was inspired by Christian and Hindu ideas such as the Body of Christ and the large body of the guru, as well as by the recognition that human exceptionalism was blinding me to my continuous and complete dependence for health and well-being on the bodies of the species, habitats, and life as a whole. Historical and archeological progress were revealing this through the recognition that urbanism has inevitably led to transformation of Edens into deserts. This was key because it allowed me to see that what was happening to birds, bees, and countless other species was also happening to me, and to my species.

∾

With a variety of new frames and constructs in my doctor's bag, and with freedom from money-based managerial thinking and endlessly intrusive technologies, I was no longer obliged to be a tool of my modern tools. And I had a research subject who was desperate to help: me. I would try to solve my problems for my own sake, and share my results with others for the sake of my yet-to-transform vocation.

I could do better by living science as Thoreau and Darwin did, in the home as well as outdoors or abroad. I could draw on the spirit of the Scottish Enlightenment that created interventionist medicine, especially its most famous brainchild Sherlock Holmes, whom Dr. Sir Arthur Conan Doyle had based on three of his professors at the University of Edinburgh medical school. I could observe life and learn from it—like the medical detectives of the great clinics of the past.

CHAPTER FIVE

The Science of
Everyday Life

――――――

S OME SAY THAT WE LIVE OUR WAY into new ideas rather than coming up with innovations that we then try to use in our lives. As I prepared to turn my personal life narrative into a detective story in the spirit of Dr. Doyle, I realized that I was already acting as a scientist and a detective, and had only to become aware that my life had become—in part—a continuing process of observation and discovery. I began to think of this process as the science of daily life, and to apply it to the whole of my life. I also became more aware of continually developing and ruling out specific hypotheses as to the causes of my ailments. In the back of my mind, I continued to rely on Occam's Razor—to recognize that it was likely that a single explanation would account for all my problems, and that I should attempt to construct one comprehensive causal theory.

I did not journal my observations, trusting that if one were important enough, I would observe it again and again, under different conditions, and allow it to change my life gradually. Some moments did stand out on their own, however.

⁓

As I began to experiment on myself, I recognized that I was using a continuous "N-of-1" study design. This empowering and potentially open-ended design was—perhaps paradoxically advocated—by Dr. Thomas Chalmers, the father of meta-analysis, and Dr. David Sackett, the father of evidence-based medicine. It has many, many advantages over all other prospective and retrospective designs, including the present gold standard—the expensive and fallible randomized, triple-blind, placebo-controlled trial used for new pills. The advantages include:

1. No outside funding needed.

2. No wait required.

3. No assumption that everyone is the same or can be grouped by known factors.

4. No assumption that whatever preoccupies the investigator or medical literature, or whatever expectations may be limiting them, are relevant to the case.

5. The study subject has the perfect control subject—that is, the intervention and control subjects are one in the same person.

6. The design controls for any number of unknown factors such as genes and modifiers of gene expression—free from the limits of statistical models that do not suit biology, medicine, or learning.

7. Responsive to new information and circumstances and thus conducive to learning. resilient to frame and construct changes and therefore conducive to ongoing evolution, knowledge, and wisdom of a suitable doctor.

8. You can—if you have enough clinical knowledge or a

doctor who is free of top-down control and possessed of ingenuity and curiosity—use and reuse this design until you solve your problems.

9. You can revise it as you form and rule out hypotheses.
10. You can focus on personal care and cure.
11. You can use it without the help of experts governed by external, arbitrary, ill-fitting, or irrelevant standards.

This study design requires the highest standard of ethical integrity on the part of the investigator-subject. You must put the truth before your preferences and habits and be ready to go against the grain. Starting with prepared, ongoing forgiveness of self and others is a must; otherwise, your personal narrative will become like the Book of Job: a key cautionary tale and no more. It also helps to develop contemplative skills: you have to think in a disciplined way and kill your own darlings, and there may be no one in your life who is willing or able to do that with you. Insight work can help you learn inner, perceptual independence of mind. Self-patterning for discovery, as per the Discovery sequence of Living Future Medicine (www.LivingFutureCourses.com), is also very helpful.

For additional self-patterning, I recommend: Maimonides' *yetzer hatov-yetzer hara* practice with embodiment of the tree of life, as per Rabbi Ted Falcon's *A Journey of Awakening*, which also builds contemplative skills; Ira Stone's *A Responsible Life*, or a local Mussar practice group, or Roger Lipsey's *Gurdjieff Reconsidered* with P. D. Ouspensky's *The Fourth Way* or a local Gurdjieff group; and the non-ideological dialogue in Marc-Alain Ouaknin's *The Burnt Book* as modified by Susan Partnow for Compassionate Listening. Platonic and Socratic dialogues are also helpful for patterning objectivity and deepening responsiveness.

Traditionally, clinicians developed disease definitions with gold standards and etiopathogeneses, as I do in this book. They also proposed hypotheses as to cause, relief, and cure. But as statistical studies gained ascendancy for the confirmation or rejection of capstone hypotheses, and expectations and criticisms of preliminary studies led to distancing from tradition, the latter ceased to hold any weight. With increasing top-down managerial control, the demand for studies that contrasted with alternative policy choices or strategies increased, and preliminary learning was relegated to the laboratory and fully decontextualized. This became a problem very quickly, as management and other social processes tend to be fixed and biology soon bypasses them.

At this point in history, discovery has been delegated and disabled. Because context is everything in medicine, the dots between context and disease are failing to connect. This is untenable. When the living context is dying of injury by humans who depend on it, it's time to engage a better choice—the N-of-1 study that may divert catastrophe by preventing needless delay.

Today's over-managed and decontextualized investigators lack the freedom and time to develop their own minds or to acquire new ways of thinking like those developing in fields such as archaeology, architecture, agriculture, and history—which are already well on the way to reframing modern problems and creating new views and constructs (see *Writing on the Wall* by Karen Stern). The investigator-subject is thus obliged to seek self-care and-cure anyway, and may as well accept the use of a disregarded but better design, the

N-of-1 study—especially in suspected cases of chronic exposure. Information can be aggregated into knowledge after the fact—with or without statistics. Life is short and the art is long—as with any living art centered on biology. Now, when the status quo has ceased to respond to context, the N-of-1 study frees the maverick to push past codependence with the problem, and to proceed directly to problem-solving. This can radically shorten the art.

$$\sim$$

Within a few months of my crash after decades of eating allergenic whole grain foods, and fourteen years of an ovolactovegetarian diet I had adopted for ethical reasons à la Thoreau, I resolved to alter all of my habits. I began by trying a little fish broth at the local sushi restaurant. As I lifted the bowl of miso to take a sip, the aroma braced me, and the sip of broth infused me with well-being. After that meal, I felt better than I'd felt for months. This gave me hope, and although I struggled with my ethics, I decided I was a *speciesist:* If it came down to me, a fish, or a non-human animal, I would put myself first. I began to eat and to cook Japanese cuisine. The family liked it, and I could get authentic imported ingredients in the international district of Seattle. I felt better on dinners of udon, sukiyaki, sashimi, rice, and fish. After going to Japan, I also enjoyed eating rice and fish for breakfast.

Over the years, I found that my well-being was affected by the cuisine, locale, and cost of the food that I ate from that point on. I did well eating in Japan, parts of New Mexico, and Italy—especially Rome, where I was able to walk all day and skip my afternoon rest. Expensive gourmet food was also easy to tolerate. I wished I could eat it every day.

This and other experiences pointed to food as a cause of my illness. I had trouble with wheat and dairy, tomatoes and potatoes, soy and corn. I began to shop carefully at the local food co-ops and farmer's markets. Then my conventional allergist discovered circulating IgG antibodies to several foods—tomatoes and stone fruit, for example. And while my physician had diagnosed leaky bowel, and its treatment had made a big difference in my life, I still had brain fog that I could only assess by doing Dell Crossword Puzzles: If I could do a five-star puzzle, I'd use the morning to write. If I could only do a two-star puzzle, I would give it up. But my neurologic symptoms did not relate to meal times; I saw no correlation between them and the foods I was eating.

In addition to changing my diet, I took careful note of my rest and activity cycles and their impact on my well-being. I would walk two miles or so a day, and sleep up to twelve hours each night. I also took a daily rest. Contemplative practices that were more restful than sleep proved very helpful, and during my rest I would often watch an inspirational or artistic film for stimulation and socialization. Over the years, I watched upwards of 3000 films, which kept me in touch with the culture and offset my isolation.

I began tracking changes in ways of thinking and acting, especially in the spiritual activism that crossed social boundaries. For a while, I did my civic duty by participating in local politics, which led me to believe that localism was the way of the future. I eventually decided to go on a news and advertising holiday and never looked back, which freed me from the media mindset and allowed me to discover what I considered to be real news.

I also observed that I felt almost normal in healthy habitats, especially in the Olympic National Park and other places that preserved remnants of the temperate rain forest. I wished I could spend more time there, but did not feel well enough. Even so, I came to see I was part of the body of my habitat and of the body of life, and that as a city dweller, I was stripped of the protection offered by my habitat.

Then I found a doctor who worked in an integrative practice and who helped me to reach a breakthrough: Dr. Fernando Vega.

Dr. Vega was like me in that he saw the big picture and used it to intervene in practical ways. But in many ways, he was even more atypical than I. His father was a scientist, a marine biologist who had taken the family to faraway places. While living in Alaska as a child, Dr. Vega had experienced the big Anchorage earthquake; in the Philippines, he had lived in the jungle. But after qualifying in family practice, renting an office, and putting up a shingle, few patients came to see him. Eventually, as a Filipino-American of Chinese extraction who was socially networked in the Asian community in Seattle, he heard of a woman who was trying to start an acupuncture practice and was persuaded to open an office with her. That practice soon took off, grew into an integrative medical clinic with dozens of practitioners of all kinds, and by the time I visited it, had flourished for more than three decades.

When I first went to see Dr. Vega, he was still using paper charts and spending as long on the intake visit as it took to get to know the patient. My appointment lasted for two hours—we didn't finish until 7 pm—at which point he said, "I think we can help you."

He gave me an elimination diet and information on how to order the liquid diet alpha-ENF™. He and his team had been collaborating with his patients, most of who were—like me—highly educated women connected with the nearby University of Washington campus. Through painstaking observation and trial and error, they had come up with an intervention that was working in our locavore economy—and that might work in others. Medicare later forced him to go digital, so his attention and concentration were temporarily—at least—diverted from medical to virtual reality, but when I met him, he was one of the few holdouts in the city who was still doing pure allopathic medicine that focused on reality and incorporated experiential learning.

In a few weeks, I was much better—and I kept getting better. But as the time came to add back more foods to improve my nutrition, I couldn't seem to find any that didn't make me sick. I stayed on the diet. I lost weight. And, after a while, I was no longer in pain. My suffering plummeted. My head cleared. I wasn't able to keep up with healthy people unless they were much older, but I had a new lease on life and was actually living my definition of a cure: the creation of a new and better life.

During this period, I helped myself along by shifting my medical detection into high gear and, like everyone else who had a project, blogged about it. I progressed step-by-step, finding the causes of my symptoms one at a time. The following redacted blog posts highlight two minor but useful discoveries.

Cure Blog, 2013, Pink Mold. After sticking strictly to the Vega diet for a few weeks, I decided to buy a bag of organic root chips containing beets that had been baked without additives.

I could eat beets, so the chips seemed like a good bet. At lunch a few days later, I grabbed a handful and ate with gusto. After the third chip, my mouth was hurting. This was not unusual, so I had another. After this chip, my mouth began to bleed. I went to look in a mirror and saw several blood blisters on my tongue and palate. As I rinsed my mouth, several of the blisters burst, bled, and kept on bleeding.

A week on, while absently biting into a pear from the refrigerator, I felt the same pain and found another blood blister. I couldn't imagine what a fresh pear and baked chips had in common, but upon taking the pear into better light and examining it closely I saw a pinkish spot in the remaining flesh at the edge of the bite—the pear was moldy.

I recalled a story from medical school to the effect that the white mold that grew on our stale, refrigerated bread was penicillium, which produced penicillin. That toxin attacked bacterial cell membranes, but had no effect on human ones. The mold I had just eaten was not like penicillium; it produced a toxin that damaged human cells. A helpful article on the internet pinpointed the pink mold as fusarium, which, when it grows naturally on foods, produces a variety of toxins.

Cure Blog, 2013, Umbilical Hernia. During a routine visit to Dr. Tracy Johanssen of Northwest Women's Health Care, she noticed that I had lost seventeen pounds since my last visit. Having been on a limited diet, and having noticed its effects, I wasn't surprised. As she asked me about it, I repeated an observation that I'd made before, which was that it seemed that I had intermittent bowel blockage. Not classic obstruction with an increase in activity and noise, but stasis, lack of forward movement with bloating and constipation.

Being quick-witted and accustomed to solving patients' problems, she suggested that I had an umbilical hernia, that is, a hernia of the belly button.

In the next week or so, I examined my belly button from time to time and found what seemed like soft masses or tense swelling, as if bits of tissue now and then protruded between my belly muscles into the navel. They felt like umbilical and peri-umbilical hernias. They went away when I lay down, but sometimes became tight and hard to reduce, to push back inside. This tended to happen after I ate foods that were rich in fats or carbohydrates, and that led to bloating.

I learned with persistence, and a small amount of discomfort, to reduce the hernia as needed. When I reduced it, many of my symptoms eased, and I could stand or sit for long periods of time rather than needing to walk or lie down. While the hernia might be small, it seemed to trap bits of soft tissue rather than lengths of bowel, and to turn my belly blank—to block the reflexes, sensations, and normal activity between my ribs and pelvic brim. Reducing the hernia eased these symptoms as well.

Now that I knew that mold or hernias might be problems, I could eliminate or mitigate them, and so reveal my underlying symptoms.

∾

Prompted by Dr. Vega, who was concerned about my nutritional needs, I redoubled my efforts to add foods to my diet list. After months of trial and error, I found that source was key: I could eat any foods, including wheat and dairy, if they were trusted single-source organics or better—with 'better' meaning purchased directly from the grower at a farmer's market after a careful conversation to ensure that the soil and crops were pristinely cared for and the produce was fresh that day.

When I recognized the pattern, I looked forward to eating bread and butter, which I missed. I couldn't wait to tell Dr. Vega. And then, as I was standing in front of the bar that divided the kitchenette from the living and dining area in the apartment that we were renting after downsizing, arms out to the side in a stretch, it hit me. The diagnosis. I had seen it before. I had organophosphate poisoning—or something just like it.

Sitting down hard on the sofa, I realized that I and every other M.D. I knew had missed the diagnosis because no one suspected it could be chronic. Or that it could result from everyday exposures. Or that it could cause continuous neurotoxicity.

As a medical student, I had seen a patient with this diagnosis who had been brought in by the police after they found him lying in the street unconscious. His drug screen was negative. He was drooling, his pupils were dilated, and he had lost control of his bladder and bowels. The resident in charge gathered all the students and residents on the ward to examine the patient and consider the signs and symptoms. Then, with a theatrical flourish, the resident injected atropine—a neurotransmitter, and in this case the antidote—into the patient's IV. The patient woke up, looked around in surprise, and soon confessed that it had become cold out on the street and he had nowhere to go. When he saw a tented house where some work was being done, he had scrambled under the yellow and black police tape and crawled inside to sleep. The problem? The house he chose had been fumigated with a pesticide "roach bomb."

That had been a mild case. Agricultural exposures could be worse, and terrorist attacks worst of all. One day, several years ago, a visiting doctor from Tokyo who was dining at our house mentioned that he had been chief resident on call at the time of the sarin subway disaster. Organophosphates were originally developed as agents of biological warfare but had, in a fit of post-WWII wishful thinking, been repurposed for agricultural and household pesticide use, and were easy to concoct. The subway incident occurred during rush hour, and quickly overwhelmed the hospital with comatose patients. Initially, they didn't know what agent had been used, but the team of house staff in charge of research soon pinpointed it. A resident injected atropine into one of the first patients to be admitted. The patient was cured. They then called for atropine from area hospitals, and most lives were saved.

But I had no known history of exposure. My case, and perhaps countless others, had to have arisen from a life that was—by the standards of the day—extremely low risk. *It must have been in my food.* I must have been eating poison every day, but not enough to lead to loss of consciousness, or death. Just enough to stay sick. I must have missed the relation to meals because I was storing it in my fat tissue, which released it between meals. I knew that I was a slow metabolizer due to Gilbert's syndrome and to at least two genes. These were probably the reason that I had a chronic neurotoxicity rather than cancer, a neurodegenerative disease, or something else. I was dumbfounded, shocked, but I understood the diagnosis there and then.

It took a week, a month, a year, and then six more years for the full implications to sink in: We humans had so baffled our species with economic models of productivity as to feed poisons to our bodies, our children, and our habitats. We had ignored warnings about DDT, pollinator death, and deterioration in human health and had stubbornly and blindly pursued a homicide-suicide attempt that looked poised to succeed. The spread of all kinds of food-related ailments had done nothing to stem the horrific and ridiculous escalation of unintentional chemical food poisoning by toxins such as organophosphorus compounds, adjuvants, Bt-producing corn and soy, and other neurotoxins synthetic or natural. We were to our technologies like toddlers to Uzis. We were a danger to self and others and worse: to the wondrous body of life that had taken 300 million years to evolve.

The world landed on my shoulders. I was aware that millions of patients might be developing epidemic ailments due to neurotoxins that threatened their habitats, and that I might be the only person in the world who grasped the full scope of the problem. The monkey was on my back, and nobody I appealed to would listen. To confirm my conclusion for myself as well as others, I proceeded to do an experiment.

Cure Blog, 2013, Corn as Poison. After I learned to avoid foods that showed any signs of mold or blight, and to reduce my umbilical hernia after eating carbs and fats, I turned again to trying new foods. At a favorite neighborhood restaurant that was not too expensive, but which served dishes that I could eat with minimal symptoms, I noticed I could not eat salads with dressing, and I began to suspect that one of the causes of my illness was vegetable oil.

Then I remembered having met a woman in a nearby

county who told me the story of her experiences with corn: She had been ill for a couple of years and had found that any kind of corn product caused her to feel sick. She had tried corn oil, corn syrup, cornstarch, and so on, and found that any and all of them could sicken her. Having experienced headache and difficulty with equilibrium, she had been told that she had migraines. She accepted this, but to me her symptoms sounded as if she might have had neurotoxicity due to pesticide poisoning.

As I paid attention to oils, I noticed now that I had problems with peripheral nerve pain and tingling when I ate foods that contained soy or corn, or derivatives of those foods, such as soy lecithin. I wondered in passing if the culprit at the restaurant was corn oil, but suspected that if it was, it was not the only one. After a bit, it seemed that canola oil might be to blame, so for a time I would ask for no canola oil when I ate out. The dishes served were often missing sauces and other added sources of flavor and, unhappily, didn't necessarily prevent toxicity.

I decided to experiment with oils. I went on a strict Vega diet and allowed my weight to return to the recent low. Then I went to a regular supermarket and bought familiar brands of canola, safflower, and corn oil. One morning, I took 1 tablespoon of canola oil. I felt a mild soreness in my throat, but otherwise nothing. I waited. Still nothing. The next day, I heated the oil to smoking, let it cool, and took 1 tablespoon of burnt canola oil. Still nothing. A few days later, I repeated the process for safflower oil with similar results.

Some days later, I took 1 tablespoon of corn oil in the morning. After noting no increase in symptoms, I took one more tablespoon of burnt oil in the afternoon. That evening, I noticed I was feeling poorly. I had a bad night. After a recovery period of more than a week, I repeated the experiment by taking ¼ cup of corn oil in the morning. Bingo. I experienced a flare of the symptoms that had first been diagnosed as chronic fatigue syndrome, then as myalgic encephalomyelitis (ME), and then as chronic Lyme disease. I never want to repeat the experiment. It was hell and it wasn't over in a hurry.

Results, beginning on the morning of 4/3/13:

8:00 am	Drank 16 oz of tea made from a blend of black and green tea leaves.
9:24 am	Took 1/4 cup conventional corn oil.
9:25 am	Sore throat.
9:50 am	Unmistakable flare with increased tingling and pain in my feet, sinking energy, difficulty concentrating, general fatigue, heart discomfort, stomach twinges, and difficulty breathing.
10:08 am	Muscle aches and tremor.
10:09 am	Brain fog; could no longer work and laid down on the couch.
10:12 am	Got up to eat turkey beet risotto per the Vega diet.
10:15 am	Irritable.
10:33 am	Laid down again.
11:04 am	Muscle fasciculations (involuntary twitches).
11:50 am	Symptoms began to ease.
12:16 am	Took a fat and alcohol challenge to the liver in the form of an ice cream sundae with a jigger of rum followed by a meal of butter and crackers (an imprecise challenge, as I later learned).

12:54 am   Worse.

1:00 pm   Hellish state with paranoia.

1:40 pm   Began tea flush with three sixteen-ounce servings.

5:10 pm   Took vitamin and protein antidote in the form of a twelve-ounce drink of water with powders from Energy Revitalization System™ and alpha-ENF™.

5:50 pm   Dinner meal per Vega diet.

6:46 pm   Distended belly; unable to reduce hernia.

7:47 pm   Nausea.

Then, on consecutive days:

4/4/13   Took spicy Ethiopian lunch challenge; worse again; some brain fog.

4/5/13   Low again; took wine, dairy, and charred foods to challenge liver; brain fog worse.

4/6/13   Bad morning; took an olive oil antidote, which may have eased catabolism of fat depots, added to abdominal fat, and reduced immediate symptoms.

∾

Proof is what it takes to convince. Given my many recurrences of toxicity in the course of reintroducing foods into my daily diet, I didn't need any more proof. And while I had been assured in the past that the effects of corn were mediated by allergy, I could no longer believe that (though I do have some food allergies which, once induced by irritants, do not go away.) I felt obligated to accept what was a very inconvenient and very unpleasant reality: Corn, the food that my great-grandfather and his ancestors had adopted generations ago from Native

American agronomists, had become a late modern poison in the context of industrial farming.

I thought of Darwin's autobiography, the part where he describes—for the benefit of his scientist children—how hard it is to see something that hasn't been seen before, even when you are looking for it and are immersed in it. That had certainly been the case for me. Since my first child was born in the late 1980s, I'd had a part in the rising rates of asthma, depression, mysterious gastrointestinal complaints, allergic reactions to food, and worsening chronic illness and disability. I had been looking to define and solve the problems that my former colleagues are to this day still trying to ignore. I had all of the education and experience I needed to identify the problem, and even more motivation—I was literally desperate. But I had missed it. Not because it was like the purloined letter, hidden out in the open, but because it was too horrifying to consider.

It didn't surprise me that the medical care delivery system was dependent on technologies that could not penetrate the unwanted and unimaginable. New information comes from the patient-doctor encounter or from the doctor patient.

But few doctors listen or indulge healthy curiosity. They are too busy looking at the computer. One of my medical school professors, Dr. Arthur Herbst, was the first to report that mothers' use of diethylstilbestrol (DES) during pregnancy put their teenage daughters at risk of a rare cancer called vaginal adenocarcinoma. What was most extraordinary about Dr. Herbst was his open mind. When his patients asked, "Do you think it could have been the DES I took during pregnancy?" He listened. Had he not been on the faculty at Harvard, and possessed of confident determination, he might not have listened even then, when he and his peers took it as their duty.

When human health is involved, there is no point in looking into mice or molecules. Clinical observations in the course of care—a process that dates back to Hippocrates at least—are the source of new knowledge of ailments. Patients and doctors who have the confidence and curiosity to question their experiences and to observe them carefully are able to identify and define phenomena that are new. The doctor is then able to draw on a lifetime of study and experience and—with luck—to name and analyze a new ailment and eventually to discern a gold standard for diagnosis. This is how clinical discoveries are made, and how problems are defined in a way that opens the door to further investigation.

Such investigation may lead to the development of confirmatory diagnostic tests that satisfy managers and that stand up in court. Eventually, a screening test may prove worthwhile. Unfortunately, and expensively, many patients and an increasing proportion of doctors imagine that technology is the source of new knowledge. Nothing could be further from the truth. All doctors and all tests make mistakes when judged against our best human comprehension. The body is infinitely complex, and our thinking is not. Our dislike of uncertainty causes us to deny or overlook the fact that too many overly-precise tests can lead to harmful over-treatment. If you want to stump your late modern doctor, ask what the positive and negative predictive values of the test are in comparison to the gold standard in patients like you. And if they are getting the test to "treat the chart," as the saying goes, consider refusing it.

Medical detection and clinical research begin with sketching a big picture that may guide us to the right details. For example, myalgic encephalomyelitis is far more common in women and tends to follow childbirth. Is this because of the massive loss of newly accumulated fat tissue and its stores of poisons? I still don't know. To my knowledge, this fact has never been used as a clue in the investigation of its causes, or its consequences.

Until we do the clinical detective work that can answer questions like these, we will be wise to put our molecular theories into perspective. Bodies may dazzle us with their myriads of molecules and their fascinating patterns of action and consequence, but to see an emerging epidemic in terms of its molecular process is like trying to comprehend the weather by watching a few droplets of moisture coalesce inside a cloud. It is more useful to watch the cloud. In medicine, that means doing the kind of clinical research that Dr. Vega had been doing, and that I had been able to take advantage of by turning my life into an N-of-1 study.

I now knew what I needed to know to help myself, and help myself I did. But I still had questions. Did my neurotoxicity derive from the chemicals applied to soils and crops? To those added later? To genetically modified organisms? To all that was done to food in the name of science? The causes weren't yet everywhere, or the elimination diet would have failed.

Was chronic poisoning causing fatty liver or cirrhosis in me? Did poisoning cause obesity and liver disease? What end stage disease or diseases may trigger late modern understanding of chronic exposure? No one knows. The clinical science isn't there yet, and standard modern methods are unlikely to provide it. Progress will depend on dissemination of the N-of-1 study, and its integration into routine clinical care, after which collection and aggregation of data may be of use.

Despite all my unanswered questions, I stopped my research there, as I didn't want to make myself ill, or to get lost in inner space.

～

I talked to everyone I knew, or could strike up a conversation with, about my work. I spoke to highly successful friends who were making up to a quarter of a million dollars a year to protect human health. I wrote to over 100 experts. I talked to my senator. But no one—except the folks at my local food co-op, who were expecting this—listened to me.

Two conversations I had when I first started ailing came back to haunt me. One was with a colleague who was working in the same sick building as I. As she walked into the building through the revolving door, her face turned beet red. I asked her about it. She didn't want to talk about it, but after some urging said that her face turned red every time she walked in the door—and stayed red until she left.

I said, "No one wants to talk about how many of us are getting sick with all kinds of things. It's like Love Canal. People are developing all kinds of diagnoses. We need to be finding a way to identify cases by causal pathways, or by exposure, like in an occupational study."

Her answer? "We'd never get funded."

"But our lives and our health are on the line!"

She looked around to make sure that no one was listening before admitting, "Our methods just don't work for this."

We shared a dark laugh at the irony of the situation: two floors of epidemiologists looking away from a disease outbreak occurring amongst us. I later found out that the building was sealed tightly to save energy, and its owners never changed the air filters. The filters had been at 50% capacity when it sold.

The other conversation was with a colleague I ran into while wrapping up my work. When I told her I was sick, that my case was part of an emerging epidemic, and that "I need somebody to be really good at our job right now," she looked at me in alarm and replied, "Well don't look at me!" Then she scurried away.

The people I knew took my pleas for help as conversation, and told me about the struggles with the work they were doing—which was, at our time in life, generally administrative work focused on the institution that employed them. There was no expression of curiosity, no concern for the future of the species. They saw themselves as doing their part in a system that was working, or would work eventually. All such conversations ended in the equivalent of a busy signal or disconnection.

Our methods don't work. But don't look at me. I'm busy.

I went into what humorist Patrick McManus calls a modified stationary panic. I freaked out.

Then I forged ahead alone. I had a vision of what I needed to do, and did my best to get there. And my methods worked. I had uncovered the cause of my illness and needed only to share that information and my futurist solutions about care and cure. Or so I thought.

CHAPTER SIX

Everything Goes to Hell

Aftera couple of years of recovery, I begantodecline—subtly and slowly, but inexorably. I blamed my deterioration on the long-term consequences of eating poisons with irritants and breathing allergens with pollutants. I upped my asthma meds. I wrote. I wondered if I would get the word out before my time was up. I thought I might be finished.

And then I experienced a crash that would cost me almost everything I hadn't lost the first time, including my sense of safety. I was frightened, but I knew this fierce grace was part of getting to the bottom of an epidemic. So I bucked up and took it as a duty and privilege to uncover a hidden hazard that I had missed before. This one seemed diabolical; it led to a form of neurotoxicity that was unnerving, sometimes even terrifying. I feared that I might have a psychotic break from which I would never recover—unless, of course, I could pinpoint and avoid the cause before that happened.

There was an "aha" moment this time, too.

One morning I was gazing out the dining room window of our condo and noticed the knob-and-tube wiring on the outer wall. The knob-and-tube style carries a unidirectional current; it does not cancel out the field it creates. It was long ago supplanted by wiring that sends current in both directions. I often sat in the dining room, writing, with my back to that window. Toward that wire. I suddenly realized, "Oh shit."

We had known the electrical system for the condo building into which we had moved three years earlier was way out of date. I realized then that I had missed a neurotoxin that had been penetrating my whole body long enough to overcome my tolerance to it. The world had become an inside-out micro-wave oven amped up by emissions across the electromagnetic spectrum. Many modernists love to hate the people who name it: non-ionizing radiation poisoning from pervasive, artificial electromagnetic fields.

Our species did not evolve for this environment.

I did not want to have to blow the whistle on this one. I knew exactly what I would be facing. To say this out loud would be to commit late modern medical and technological heresy. The fact that it would be obvious in retrospect would be of no help for years, probably the rest of my life. You see, my first faculty job had been in the department where Nancy Wertheimer had taken a Master of Science in Public Health. She was an independently wealthy woman who took that degree in order to study the relation between step down electrical transformers and neighborhood childhood cancer. She had found higher odds of exposure in cancer cases, and had published her finding with statistician Ed Leeper. This was the first report of a harmful effect of non-ionizing radiation in a human population.

All hell broke loose. The power industry was outraged, then offered funding to researchers in the hopes of countering her findings. This is typical of epidemiology when it impinges on a sensitive topic: The cart is put before the horse. The unavoidable sociopolitical aspect of this very new and seat-of-the-pants specialty pushes the science into a closet and slams the door on it. Because life is risky and habits resist change, there is overwhelming pressure to bow to the status quo when things get rough—unless risk is extreme, predictable, and terrifies the complacent. People who work in public health are used to this, and practice their art under the guidance of politicians because politics is the art of the possible, and so is public health. It depends on social consensuses that are slow to change.

This shouldn't, in theory, affect the ivory tower, but it does. In such cases, policy studies may be done before the necessary groundwork is laid. In other words, applications leap ahead of theory, and panic is "treated" by reassurances before the truth can be learned. Absent high death rates, rapid spread, and comprehension, it is more feasible for authorities to play down the problem and to allow scapegoating of the sick than to face an angry public that has little or no respect for the unknown.

And sadly, researchers follow money and status. In my department—Nancy Wertheimer's department—this happened immediately. A mentor of mine did a state-of-the-art study that would, in retrospect, make a great cautionary tale for use in the training of Epidemics Intelligence Service officers. It seemed to have been designed to conceal any and all hazards of exposure, and so to bury rather than uncover the truth.

Like Dr. Sam Milham, a one-time state epidemiologist who conjectured online as to how dirty electricity may cause cancer, my mentor viewed exposures arbitrarily and post-hoc—sometimes years later. He did so in the absence of clinical observations that might allow investigators to take a wild guess as to how to assess radiation dose when studying a particular outcome. No one had worked out what timing, duration, or power of radiation in what electromagnetic frequency ranges might do harm to what tissues, or what ailments might result. Having thus guessed at exposure during a time when exposure was skyrocketing, the study found nothing, and investigators concluded that there was nothing to find. That was the wrong conclusion. In such a case, finding nothing means nothing, proves nothing. It's a waste of money that does great harm.

When I challenged him on his exposure assessment back then, he said, "The utility guys shouldn't take the blame if people want to use personal electrical or electronic devices."

Like stereotypical bureaucrats, utility workers thought from an organizational perspective; they persuaded my mentor that the issue was the mothers' angst, and that it was unfair to point the finger of blame at them.

This obscures a reality: from a biological perspective, social views are irrelevant. A valid assessment must be biologically meaningful as well as accurate, reliable, and complete. The same is true for assessment of the consequences. There is no reason to believe that cancer is the outcome of greatest concern. The fact that time and money have been spent on many studies that found nothing proves nothing, but reinforces complacency. This is unfortunate, and tells us more about the blind spots of late modern thinking than about the health consequences of late modern radiation.

Nancy Wertheimer, who spent years of her time and a small inheritance to do a study in simpler times, used modern methods when they were still valid—which was before exposure had become ubiquitous, high-dose, and long-term. She *had* found something—and was, according to her obituary, publicly attacked by utility companies for the rest of her life.

Attacks were the last thing I needed, and I knew that was what I would get, too. The internet and comedians only help to shore up public conceit. Everyone knows to ridicule the guy wearing a metal colander for a hat. The Rhys Darby character in Taika Waititi's film *Hunt for the Wilderpeople* is a classic example of this stereotype. The character is funny, and audiences seem to take successful satire as evidence of biological truth.

So, my threshold for accepting this unwelcome reality was very high. The stigma would make my life very, very difficult. Everyone would think I was nuts. And, in a way, I was. If I or any of my colleagues had paid more attention to the limitations of our studies, and spoken out more often, this might not have happened. But it had, and I could not escape it. My body was in trouble. The good news was that I could, once again, do better. I could try to help myself, at least.

As with the "aha" moment that led to my understanding of the role of chemical food poisoning in my case of "chronic fatigue," this one had a lead-up.

Around six months earlier, I noticed that I was having trouble writing, in the old way—my head was fuzzy. My reaction times were slower. I needed twice as much afternoon rest time. It's easier to see all of this in retrospect. At the time, I accepted the familiar. It wasn't until I had new symptoms—unusual ones, like dark, blank thoughts—that I became concerned.

Because wild habitats had always relieved my symptoms, I wanted to live in it or near enough to it to walk in it as needed. I thought about moving from Seattle to San Juan Island, so

I rented a house in the fall to try it out, planning to stay the winter. The house was big. The owners had built it themselves. It was at the top of a bluff above the Salish Sea, on a hill next to a University of Washington research facility that had 200 acres of forest where I could go walk. The air was clean. It seemed perfect.

After settling in, though, I noticed there was no ventilation in the house, and that this seemed to affect the air quality. The gas heating stove in the middle of the house smelled bad, as did the electrical wall heating units which had been set directly into the log walls. I thought perhaps the air was impure, and neurotoxic.

I stuck it out. After Thanksgiving, I noticed that when I sat alone at the dinner table at night, I had very dark thoughts. It's hard to describe. It was different than being depressed. It was like walking into the pages of a dark urban fantasy in which I was the last person alive and had no reason to live, and was a big blank inside like the open mouth in the horror film called *The Ring*, or a character in a recent play by Ruth Ozeki.

I would get up and write. Or put on music. Or call someone. Or knit. Or watch a movie. Nothing made it better. And for the first time, writing made it worse. It was like walking into a horror movie, but it wasn't titillating—it was numbing. Daylight made things better—as did walking in the forest—but every night was bad. I had a little wine to induce my liver enzymes, but that only made it worse.

I thought it might be the gas heat; I had turned the central heating off in the Seattle condo unit, and that had helped. Here, it didn't. All I could do was to escape in my car.

When I got home to Seattle, wistful for the woods and the

glorious scenery of the ferry ride, I asked my husband to rent a van and pick up my things. He kindly agreed. But neither of us knew how sick *he* was. Two years earlier, he had been in the intensive care unit with sepsis and had had a systolic blood pressure of fifty for a few days. He had nearly died, and had not been the same since. When he got back from retrieving my things, his foot was dragging. We thought his boot sole was coming apart. He ignored it. But when he finished a major project and relaxed, he realized that he was in trouble and went to the emergency room where they discovered an intracranial subdural bleed. He underwent neurosurgery, with placement of a plate in his head.

When he was out of surgery and in the ICU, our daughter and I slept in his room. The hospital had high levels of non-ionizing radiation, and as I became weaker and weaker, I attributed that to stress.

When we got home, though, I started having weird problems. I had trouble sleeping. And I had terrible nightmares. Just horrific. I dreamt of being stabbed over and over by men shouting "Kill! Kill! Kill!"

We were sleeping on a latex mattress very close to the old knob-and-tube wiring, with my husband's new iPhone 6 on the nightstand. In hindsight, I can see that I was developing non-ionizing radiation poisoning with loss of tolerance, but I didn't realize it at that point. I was aware that the phone was a problem. I soon took to turning off the wi-fi when I wasn't using it, and to keeping my older iPhone off for long periods of time.

Even so, my symptoms kept getting worse and weirder. I couldn't make sense of them. I experienced optical phenomena, especially while lying in bed on my back. I saw lights, snowy images like old television shows, and hallucinatory colors; I realized that these were worse in the area opposite the place where my head had gone through the windshield during a motor vehicle accident in my college years—the area of the contracoup impact! Then I began to notice that when I walked along the sidewalk by a neighboring apartment building, it felt as if the vitality at the back of my head had been scraped away. A New Ager might say that part of my aura was gone, but my guess was that the old head injury was complicating my symptoms.

I began to have conversations in my head that were different than usual. I lost all sense of coincidence. Though my work was integrative—I had taken it upon myself to connect things that had not been connected—this was different. This was everything. I knew that I was having cognitive symptoms, including ones that I had once seen as psychotic. As a medical detective, I viewed them as symptoms of some underlying cause, and knew that I had to use what rationality I had left to find the cause before I was no longer able.

One night, I went to a guitar concert at Benaroya Hall. I was feeling tense. As I walked past a side corridor at the end of which I could see a blue light—perhaps a security system of some kind—I felt my energy body go haywire. I had done energy work when neurotoxic and had felt my core fall apart like a stack of Jenga blocks, but this was different. It was like a red alert. It felt as if my energy body might fracture along a curved surface inside the back of my left ribcage, never to unite again.

Fortunately, as I moved beyond the corridor, my symptoms eased.

I also began to see bright white light in my field of vision while I was writing, and to have difficulty with attention and concentration. I would have to stop and go lie down until it stopped. I self-diagnosed temporal lobe epilepsy, which some writers struggle with.

Not long after, I had the "aha" moment. I was standing between the living and dining rooms in the condo. I looked out the back window at the old knob-and-tube wiring. I looked around at the Blu-Ray player, out-of-region DVD player, and the large LED screen; at the walls filled with knob-and-tube wiring; at the electric space heaters I was using; at my iPhone, iPad, and MacBookPro. I would have to give them all up, along with our cutting-edge electrical appliances. I had always been an early adopter, and now I had to bail.

I knew that I had to leave the condo as well. With the rapid proliferation of wi-fi around the condo, it was becoming more and more toxic. My life had broken again. My life would never be the same. This time it was terrifying—I had no way of knowing if this form of neurotoxicity would be reversible. My rationality was eroding fast, and I had failed to find a safe place to go.

At least I could observe my responses to non-ionizing radiation poisoning. I could look for help. I could develop a working hypothesis to help me avoid exposure. I could try to detox, though I later found it would take years—more even than it had taken to clear my system of ingested neurotoxins. And I quickly learned that it was almost impossible to identify or define any particular source with accuracy or certainty. It wasn't going to be easy.

During this period, I was still looking for places where life would be healthier and easier. Bellingham seemed to be a possibility, so early that summer I went up to stay in a tiny house that a retired couple had built on an acre lot outside of town where they lived. They had created a "glamping" area on the property as well.

I had no devices. There were no cell towers nearby. There were trees on the property. I slept beautifully. The man who had built this particular tiny house had also been the president of the electrician's union, and had created a very comfortable structure. In hindsight, I can see why. Electrical errors are a big source of radiation, and of consequent health problems. The tiny house was free of those errors.

We took another trip to Bellingham, during which I became aware that radio towers were giving me problems, as was the dock of the Alaska Ferry. I don't know what the terminal emitted—perhaps marine radar?—but I couldn't be within half a mile of it or in any of the surrounding cafés or bookstores. When I was, I would experience what I can only describe as extremely unpleasant psychic pain, with a feeling of heaviness and an urge to lie down. And with it, my mood would darken.

It was like what had happened in the house on San Juan Island.

I asked a consultant to come and assess the electromagnetic radiation in the condo. The wires under the eaves gave off high readings in the bedroom upstairs and in a corner of the dining room below it. Emissions from the inner wall below the stairs were lower. The consultant was a retired satellite engineer who had bought his meters when his pregnant daughter wanted to buy a home located next to an array of high voltage electrical wires. He had used the meters to dissuade her. After that, he consulted for people who believed they were exposed to electromagnetic fields in the home.

Interestingly enough, while his intention had been to reassure them, he instead found himself confirming their concerns, as when he consulted for a woman who pointed out a harmful field several feet from the corner of her bedroom. Although he said there could be no field there, his measurements confirmed the presence of dirty electricity, and while he still trusted his meters over anyone's self-report, he had now discovered that some people were much more sensitive than his meters. A later consultant recommended a home level of one milligauss or less for someone like me. Our whole condo was well above that.

What meters fail to detect are the biological consequences of non-ionizing radiation; they also miss all other sources of toxicity. And, no meter is more accurate than my symptoms—but as detectors, my symptoms have limits. I am not a meter. Microwave towers give me an intense headache, usually after a delay. Cell phones and wi-fi do the same—until I go above a certain threshold of toxicity. The more neurotoxic I am, the less I feel. The warning symptoms go away when I need them most.

The nervous system isn't a machine. It doesn't give immediate feedback. There's no one-to-one correspondence between radiation and neurotoxicity. Something is altered deep in the brain, and manifests after a delay with some spectrum of ill-defined consequences, including insomnia. Even so, and even though my toxicity from non-ionizing radiation was becoming critical, it seemed to me that extremely low frequencies disrupted sleep, and that very low frequencies caused symptoms like organophosphorus poisoning, minus the peripheral neuritis. Our brains, which did not evolve to cope with human-created poisons, respond with dysfunctions that may be surprising, and all over the map—especially when buffeted by multiple hazards that only begin to ease in an untouched, primal forest with clean food, air, and water.

As I continued to deteriorate, I became more and more aware of my toxicity and of sources of radiation. One summer day, I went on a short walk through our densely-populated inner-city neighborhood in Seattle's Capitol Hill. As I approached a large radio tower on Madison, I felt extraordinarily heavy, as if I were suddenly moving 1,000 pounds instead of 140. It was hard to keep going, but improved as I approached the bottom of the tower. The field was not uniform, and it was weaker at the base. A friend with a strong background in physics and math confirmed that fields are not generally uniform or predictable, which made me better able to jump the gap between college physics and the real world, and so to detect exposures and antidotes. After a time, I was able to confirm my hunch that biomass (e.g. healthy forest habitat) provided good protection.

By the time I became troubled by my neighbors' automatic downloads at four or five a.m., I was in desperate need of a vacation that would take me out of the condo. I left, but the trip turned out to be harrowing; I couldn't find places free of wi-fi and cell phones. My husband insisted on using his. He was getting angrier and angrier with me. He insisted that I take high-dose anti-psychotic medication, which I tried but stopped because it made me feel much worse. When we finally got to the rental unit in Ashland, Oregon, which was far less toxic and a tremendous relief, I knew that I had to stay. He responded by ridiculing me and running away. I felt bad for him, but chose to protect myself by staying. Abandonment at that moment was the worst thing to happen in all my years of illness. It revived my secondary PTSD after a long period of recovery, and undermined my faith in the species.

I persuaded Dr. Vega—who wanted to try natural remedies—to write me a prescription for sertraline, which had eased my depression in the 90s. The very first pill helped, which isn't supposed to happen. My serotonin levels must have been close to zero. I kept the bottle of anti-psychotic pills in case I didn't get better—in case I might decide to overdose. Once again, I wasn't sure that I could continue, but I managed to keep at it. Through the fall and winter, I took walks in nature, where I often felt relief. I tried various interventions. And I observed my symptoms closely.

Very gradually, the nightmares diminished. The boundaries between sleep and waking, between dreaming and thinking, reemerged. It was as if the temporoparietal areas of the brain—or whatever was responsible for processing and indexing memories at night—were beginning to function properly again. And after I bought a house where I could turn the electricity off at the circuit breakers, and could otherwise reduce my exposure, I began to recover. Over a year after my nightmares began, I looked forward to going to bed again. Sleeping was no longer a horror.

I resumed my life.work, but as I became experienced with trying to detect exposure, I also became aware that the minute I focused on a symptom, my attention would alter my observation. In non-ionizing radiation sickness, attention is like the placebo effect—except that it may cloak rather than relieve symptoms. When I pay attention to a symptom, it becomes vague, general, and nonspecific. Even now, I have little ability to detect or to monitor my neurotoxicity. When I feel bad or have trouble sleeping, I get out into nature or stay in my one safe place: my house. When I feel tired or blue, I cut back on exposure by staying home.

I was fortunate to land in Ashland, where New Agers recognize that we are in a time of epochal change, and where other patients with my condition have diagnosed themselves and have gotten the word out. One woman—wife of a prominent local architect who has designed homes for wealthy people with my condition—also has a degree in public health, has worked with local children whose diets were toxic, and herself has had non-ionizing radiation sickness. As a result of their activism, and the work of the founders of Eco-Nest who follow the building biology paradigm, there are local tradesmen who are now aware of the issue, and who are kind and able to help. Interestingly, that woman—like other fellow patients who I've met as far away as Australia—has Puritan and pioneer roots similar to my own, which leads me to wonder if some inbreeding among the early "Yankees" may have led to a genetic predisposition.

Radiation sickness will not be going away anytime soon. Humanity is living in a self-created toxic soup of chemicals and radiation, and some of us are the early warning system for what the rest of us will eventually experience. People with the new epidemics are the canaries in the coal mine that is our post-modern environment. We may not see the effect that we are having on trees for a hundred years because that's how long they take to respond.

And we are avoiding the questions of what to do about device addiction, and all the other adverse consequences of ubiquitous electronic devices—such as how to handle the toxic solid waste they create.

Taken together, the repercussions of electric and electronic devices to life on Earth are likely to be catastrophic. They could even cause the end of all species, including ours—unless, when biology gives us the choice, "your money or your life," we choose life.

Unless we make changes now.

CHAPTER SEVEN

Alderman Syndrome

A S A MEDICAL STUDENT, I had wanted to make last-minute saves unnecessary by preventing disease, or reversing it, before potentially irreparable damage could be done. As a young academic studying causation, I learned to move back through the causal web from structural damage to early causes. That meant letting go of the modern gold standard for diagnosis: anatomy. My body taught me to identify primary causes of illness in those predisposed to show some kind of organ system dysfunction before evincing end organ damage. I was able to realize the potential of preventive medicine by discerning and defining chronic exposures that could be clinically cured by removing their causes. That is, in effect to create a preventive cure.

I am calling my condition Alderman syndrome, or chronic ambient poisoning. If you have a condition like mine, you may be able to use this actionable diagnosis to cure yourself of ongoing exposure. If it works for enough people, we may become part of a grassroots movement that reverses the tide of emerging ailments expressed by all species in various ways, and so prevent human extinction.

Our species has been the main cause of all recent extinctions —losses of individual species that are foreshadowing the sixth great extinction. We have, so far, believed so much in human exceptionalism as to remain unaware of the elephant in the room: our disregard for life. We continue our galloping consumption of habitats, as well as our poisoning of the body of life and its host planet. While our species has always fouled the nest, moderns have done so to a far greater extent and with unprecedented efficiency and self-absorption.

Medical doctors, who have been integrated into the epochal paradigm of every era in recorded history, have become embedded in the modern paradigm and have yet to recognize that they may be doing more harm—and causing more suffering and death to all life—than they can presently see. They also lack the freedom or agency to think or respond wisely, or to follow the lead of fields that are better led and less over-managed. A revival of grassroots clinical research and in-depth case studies can alleviate this problem and help to join medicine with the living paradigm that has been developing in agriculture, architecture, and other fields.

To put this in the kind of modern terms that have been passing for science, it seems that our ineffective efforts to implement solutions could be summed up—tongue-in-cheek—as: (Naïve Management of the Unknown and Incomprehensible) x (Complex Systems x Statistical Elaboration) x Analysis = Codependence with Blind Assumptions and Fatal Errors = Catastrophe.

It is clear to me that centralization and imposed helplessness are deepening the problem. What we need is a grassroots movement like the hygiene movement but informed by the rights movements of the past century, and by the movement toward personal responsibility. This is already happening, as described in Paul Hawken's book *Blessed Unrest*, and in some TED talks.

~

It is essential that clinical researchers turn their attention and ingenuity to forming an emerging paradigm for medicine that emphasizes new ideas and methods. One reason for this is that standard late modern methods cannot address chronic ambient poisoning for reasons such as the following:

Exposures Can't Be Assessed. Because many important hazards are ubiquitous, cumulative, and modified by the body, we cannot assess exposure after the fact. Worse, we are guessing as to what dose of which hazard may correlate with which ailments. Does peak dose matter? Frequency? Cumulative dose? Combined doses? We don't know; we guess. Then we gather data on our guess, and if we find nothing, conclude that there is no effect. In other words, we over-interpret the negative study and glean false reassurance.

Unexposed Groups Are Disappearing. If you collect data on a hazard and an ailment in a group of people, you can then divide them into four groups: those who have the ailment or don't, and, within each group, those who have been exposed or not. The result is a fourfold table:

AILMENT	EXPOSED	
	Yes	No
Yes	a	b
No	c	d

The odds ratio estimates the degree to which a and d dominate: ad/bc. If everyone is exposed to the hazard, you get everyone divided by no one. You get nonsense. If you break exposure into categories, you may have no one who is normal enough to be deemed unexposed, and little important spread across the other categories.

Significance Is Determined by Sample Size. If you have enough study subjects, your estimates—however modest—will turn out to be statistically "significant." This is like a popularity contest: A hot proposal that gets big funding will be able in the end to claim validation by fact of size alone. That is—tongue firmly in cheek: Big Data = Little Importance + Opportunities for Confirmation Bias. You can "prove" any number of contradictory findings.

Clinical Science is Missing. Clinicians are no longer learning from life. If you're afraid to reveal the truth in a medical record (e.g. to record legally embarrassing phrases like "I don't know," "haven't got a clue," "No idea what's going on here," "all I can do here is try to stop the patient's complaining," or "this patient is not capable of comprehending simple instructions; meth addict? illiterate? brain damage?"), your record will document a virtual reality that obscures and erodes clinical acumen. Lawyers need cases; doctors need truth and integrity.

If you're afraid to say "I don't know" in your own mind, you shouldn't do research. You won't engage the unknown openly, try and find out what's going on, or develop a new gold standard. Forget about defining a diagnosis or discerning the etiopathogenesis. Your best effort will be no more than full-price, useless folly à la the Emperor's new clothes.

If your experience is insufficient to delineate a causal web that features twenty interacting factors, you're not ready for a 'big' study. If you do use statistics be aware that the thin and fragile foundation of Popperian logic, which supports testing the null hypothesis, makes no sense in real complex systems where context is key. Also, quantitative proof will be robust only when you study risk factors that account for an overwhelming proportion of cases of rare conditions—i.e. to problems of little of no present import.

The Fallacy of Molecularism. For decades there has been a hot molecule or set of molecules that everyone wants to research; right now, it's genes. When poisons are ubiquitous, the genes that determine the kind of harm those poisons do—the common variations in enzymes that break down one or more poisons, or that make one or more end organs susceptible—come to the foreground of our attention. This would only make sense if poisons were essential and genes a matter of choice, or if the many genes that make a difference could be grouped in some useful way. Researching this would be fascinating but would not obviate the need for a better option.

These and other points, when carefully considered, add up to the good news that we humans can stop using our present ideas and methods; they are outdated and have baffled us. They were good first efforts that deserve to evolve, as I have evolved through my experience. The fields of medicine and public health are likewise ready to evolve into forms that can solve current problems.

~

What does doing better look like? We've already looked at integration over history and geography; a new view of the body and the bodies in which it nests; and the N-of-1 study that anyone can use—with the aid of a doctor researcher who can make clinical diagnoses and help to discern etiopathogeneses well prior to autopsy. Let's go back and look at some of the guiding lights of late modern medicine, some or all of whom get little attention in this upside-down time when data trumps wisdom. All of them seeded the emerging paradigm in medicine.

As far back as the 1960s, laboring away on the other side of the iron curtain, Dr. A. R. Luria was writing long narrative case studies that inspired the life work of Dr. Oliver Sacks—studies that took the medical detective genre of Berton Roueché (who originally published his stories in *The New Yorker* from 1947 to 1988) into the realm of deep narrative comprehension of complex phenomena.

In 1969, Dr. David Sackett, the father of evidence-based medicine, founded the first Department of Clinical Epidemiology at McMaster University. His colleagues' innovative medical education methods employed the case study, as in law or business—a significant departure for medicine.

Related to this was a new type of intervention study designed for individual use called the N-of-1 study. While its potential for hypothesis generation and causal narrative creation has barely been tapped, a narrative published in 2016, *n of 1* illustrates how patients like Glenn Sabin (who was diagnosed with Chronic Lymphocytic Leukemia) can help themselves when they engage grassroots traits of pioneering independence, self-reliance, personal responsibility, and a can-do attitude.

In 1973, Dr. Mervyn Susser published a book, *Causal Thinking in the Health Sciences*, that introduced ecological ideas into epidemiology research. Unfortunately, his methods were limited by excessive reliance on statistical methods, which still define publication standards. In 1988, Dr. Alvan Feinstein pointed out that such simplistic methods lack biomedical validity when used to assess the hazards of everyday life. He also castigated doctors for looking to experts in other fields like economics to solve systemic problems, such as rising costs.

Around the same time, radiologists who studied expert decision-making were applying to medicine the work of Nobel Prize-winning psychologists Amos Tversky and Daniel Kahneman. In 2005, Malcolm Gladwell featured the first application of medical decision analysis to triage at Cook County hospital (for more, see Chapter Four of Gladwell's book *Blink*). And so, a handful of individuals—some influential—recognized and illuminated modern problems that had been disregarded.

Formal recognition of the role of capable patients in developing the emerging paradigm is critical across the spectrum from the doctor-patient encounter to research policy formation. Their primary care physicians can help by engaging my books and courses.

∾

It may seem counterintuitive that illness is not expressed uniformly, but a brief examination will reveal that this is always true. For example, smoking does not always cause heart disease or lung cancer, and infection by tubercle bacilli does not always cause consumption. The expression of every illness will be modified by many factors specific to its host and environment. If illnesses affected everyone to the same degree and in the same way, there would be no need for diagnosis, and no diagnostic ambiguity.

When it comes to Alderman syndrome, a great many factors may influence the degree of poisoning at any given time; a great many more influence the consequences of chronic poisoning over time. This complexity is typical of biological systems and accounts for the difficulty in detecting patterns that relate exposure and outcome—unless the problem is caused by a new medication or change in an infectious agent that dominates the picture. In the case of recurrent poisoning by agricultural poisons in food, the signs and symptoms are strongly modified by the dose and composition of the poison cocktail; the milieu in the gut; the state of the liver; the immune response; and the storage of toxins in fat. Thus, the causal model of Alderman syndrome in any given patient must account for the possibility of a five-way interaction at the very least.

The Poison Cocktail. Being inclusive in exposure definition can add clarity when factors are additive or multiplicative in time, or are cumulative over time. I propose that we aim to sum up poison exposure in time as well as over time. Each measurement includes factors that precede ingestion of poison or follow the circulation of poisons in the blood. An example of the former is the addition of poisons with food preparation; an example of the latter is the sensitivity of an end organ that expresses signs and symptoms of poisoning.

Whenever you eat conventional food produced by modern industrial agriculture, you ingest a cocktail of poisons that includes herbicides, pesticides, and their residues, as well as genetically programmed toxins. We could have anticipated this by pausing to reflect on the potentially fatal impact of such chemicals on the workers who apply them. When more people realize this, they will be amazed that moderns should be so subject to wishful thinking and take nature so much for granted as to believe that ingesting such poisons would have no adverse effect on men, women, children, and the unborn. Only those who fixate on known pathogens and deny all other hazards could poison food—and ages-old soil—by way of preserving it.

As the resistance of crop pests increases, the levels of poisons increase, and genetically modified organisms (GMOs) increase them even more. Other sources of poison also come into the mix. These may be inhaled, as with sulfur dioxide; absorbed, as with solvents; or taken voluntarily, as with use of prescription or recreational drugs, or familiar over-the-counter addictive products such as alcohol and tobacco. They may also penetrate the body as radiation. Factors such as the wide dissemination of agricultural poisons—through pervasive derivatives, the ubiquity of additional poisons, and the protean nature of the poison cocktail that is continually delivered—could obscure and thus delay recognition of its deleterious acute and chronic effects.

The Gut. The gut is one of the black boxes of modern medicine—it's dark, low in oxygen, inaccessible, complex, and poorly known. When you ingest poisons, they may damage your gut directly and cause symptoms such as indigestion, which you may suppress with over-the-counter or prescription medication. When damage to the gut lining is severe, you may develop leaky bowel syndrome, in which the contents of the gut pass through the gut-blood barrier into the bloodstream and cause vague, flu-like symptoms due to circulation of antigens and the resulting immune response.

Ingested poisons may also attack the microbiome, that is, the good bacteria on the lining of your gut, lungs, and skin that protect you. You receive your microbiome from your parents as a baby, and further strengthen it—perhaps—later in life. If your parents' microbiome is weak, you grow up in an obsessively clean home, you rarely come into contact with healthy soil, or you take antibiotics, the microbiome in your gut may be susceptible to poisons.

The effect of ingested poisons on the microbiome is that they impair its ability to detoxify poisons, digest food, or make nutrients that you need to sustain a sanguine mood, clear mind, and healthy body. A weak microbiome is subject to imbalance and overgrowth by yeast and other bothersome organisms, as well as increased risk of familiar diseases such as typhoid fever.

The old word for feces is "night soil." This reminds you that what lives in your gut is continuous with the soil of your habitat—and can be no healthier. In the long run, the only way to keep your microbiome healthy is to heal your body with its habitat by preserving clean agricultural lands and pristine wilderness, and by playing your part in restoring and enhancing all of the interconnected habitats of the planet.

The Liver. Your liver constantly produces a responsive, ever-changing array of enzymes that may be induced by many factors, such as alcohol use, and that metabolize the toxins in your blood. Depending on your enzymes and the toxins in your bloodstream, the breakdown products of the toxins that you ingest may be more or less toxic to you than the originals. Biochemists and molecular biologists have studied these enzymes and their induction and actions.

Your microbiome and liver enzymes may detoxify all of the poisons you ingest, or your end organs may be insensitive to them. If so, you may escape signs and symptoms of illness. If the poisons overwhelm your microbiome, liver enzymes, and end organ insensitivity—as is likely with those chemicals developed for use as agents of biological warfare—you will experience signs and symptoms of poisoning that may elude diagnosis. These may change with secular or local trends in agricultural practices such as use of specific chemicals, and with your intake of liver enzyme-inducing substances such as alcohol and tobacco.

The Immune System. Early in life, your immune system learned to recognize food and to avoid responding to it. But this learning may be undone when you change your diet or your gut flora, or ingest poisons that catalyze food intolerances and allergies. Poisons cause allergies when they act as adjuvants, that is, as irritants that induce or increase the immune response. Poisons may thus cause complex symptoms by damaging the gut lining and inducing immunity and auto-immunity, as well as by causing direct toxicity and eventually permanent damage to end organs such as the nervous system.

Fat Stores. When fat-soluble poisons circulate in the bloodstream, fat tissues take them in and store them. The fat stores then release them with the fats they release between meals, overnight, or during exercise. Releasing all of the poisons from fat stores is best done slowly, over a long period of time, and should be done in combination with restoration of the micro-biome and affected end organs.

Investigating Your Own Case. If you expect that you or someone you are caring for may be affected by chronic poisoning, an N-of-1 study—like the one reported in this book—can be diagnostic as well as a guide to preventive cure or at least to helpful treatment. The annotated graphical summaries of Alderman syndrome in Figures 1 and 2 on the pages that follow may be of use to you. Elimination of a source of poison in the course of an N-of-1 trial is currently the only way to detect the adverse effect of any ubiquitous toxin (see www.LivingFutureCourses.com for online courses in cure and discovery).

The Big Picture. The new, seemingly silent, and insidious epidemics, an unknown portion of which are caused by chronic ambient poisoning, are injuries to the body of life as well as to the individual, and thus resemble infectious agents with multiple host species, or injuries such as global warming, radiation releases, and environmental catastrophes. The Bhopal chemical release, the Gulf of Mexico oil spill, recent wars, and habitat destruction due to "development" that constitute a *de facto* war on life are local consequences of the new pervasive threats to life that cannot be avoided anywhere on earth. These threats are planetary in scale and caused by modern ways of living, yet remain invisible to the modern mind because they exceed the bounds of modern perceptions—and so elude care and cure.

Opening the perceptual filter and becoming aware of

Determinants of
Poison Dosage in Time

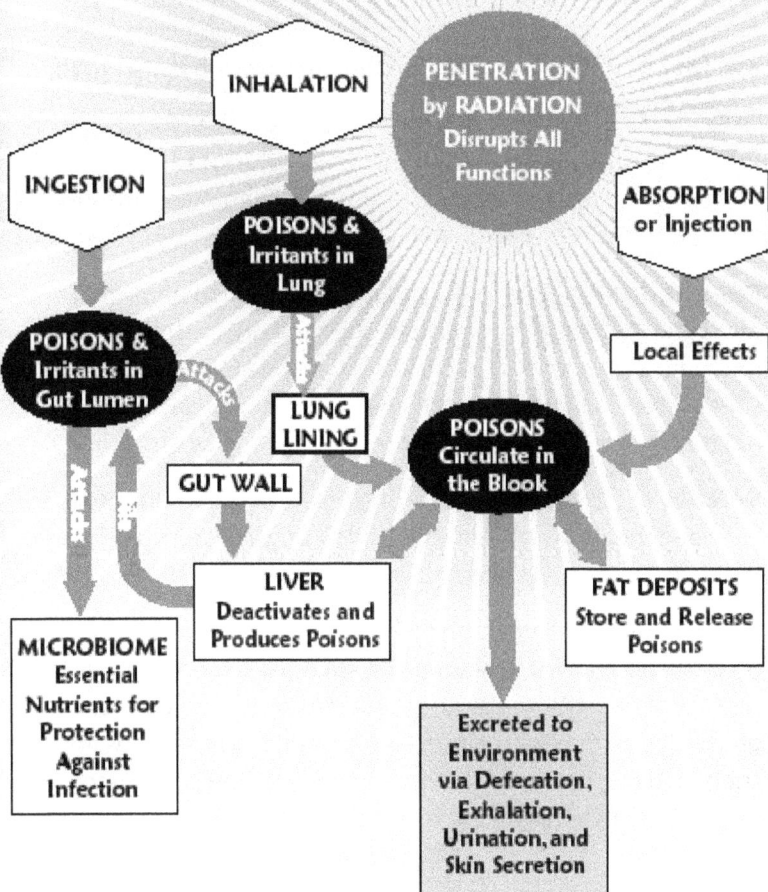

Figure 1: Diagram of Poison Intake and
Metabolism in Alderman Syndrome

Key to Figure 1

Ingestion of food, drink, and substances contaminated by man-made chemicals from sources such as: agricultural herbicides, pesticides, or genetically engineered toxin-producing organisms; animals husbanded with antibiotics, hormones or chemicals in their feed, dips, sprays, pastures, or structures; foods preserved or processed with chemicals; and foods contaminated in cooking, as through use of high temperature oils.

Inhalation of air contaminants due to spontaneous or human-produced chemicals such as volcanic ash, smoky fires, or sulfur dioxide.

Penetration by non-ionizing radiation that may damage any or all biological processes, each likely in proportion to: cumulative dose at each wavelength summed across a specific range of wavelengths; peak exposures; and susceptibility factors such as prior poisoning by a "sick structure".

Release of stored fat-soluble poisons with catabolism (e.g. between meals, overnight, prolonged physical activity, fasting, starvation, hyperthyroidism, etc.).

Circulation in blood and bodily fluids of levels that depend on intrinsic and extrinsic factors such as: genes and gene regulation; nutritional status; circulatory fitness; efficiency of excretion; recent exposure to inducers of gene expression such as alcohol, cigarettes, etc.; and past medical history (including intrauterine experiences).

Consequences of
Chronic Ambient Poisoning Over Time

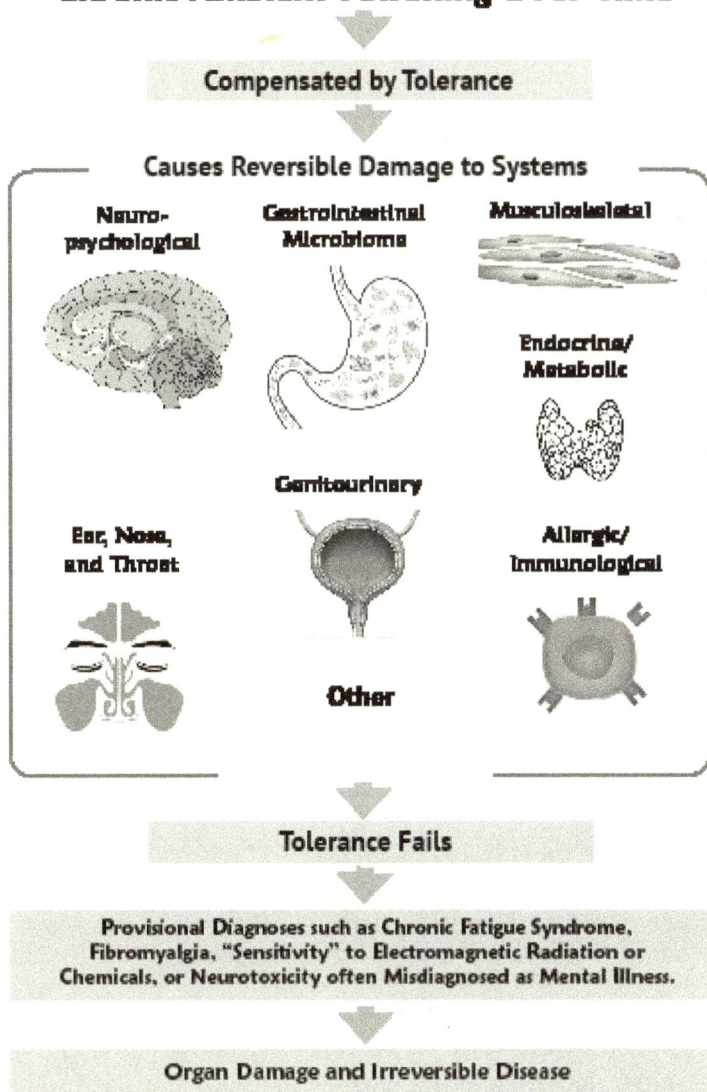

Compensated by Tolerance

Causes Reversible Damage to Systems

Neuro-psychological

Gastrointestinal Microbiome

Musculoskeletal

Endocrine/ Metabolic

Genitourinary

Ear, Nose, and Throat

Allergic/ Immunological

Other

Tolerance Fails

Provisional Diagnoses such as Chronic Fatigue Syndrome, Fibromyalgia, "Sensitivity" to Electromagnetic Radiation or Chemicals, or Neurotoxicity often Misdiagnosed as Mental Illness.

Organ Damage and Irreversible Disease

Figure 2: Diagram of Consequences of Poisoning Over Time.

Examples of Consequences (Signs, Symptoms, and Labels) in Variants of Alderman Syndrome

NERVOUS SYSTEM
Central: Confusion; loss of focus and ability to multi-task (brain fog); disorientation to time and place; failure to form new memories; periodic anomia with word substitution and loss of language fluency; circumlocution and tangential and garrulous speech; spatial confusion with loss of map-reading ability and facial recognition; tremors; tipping or falling to one side; inability to walk straight with eyes closed; loss of automatic adjustment to flow of traffic; disruption of thirst, hunger, and/or satiety with dehydration and/or weight change; pseudo-herpetic mouth ulcers, exaggerated sense of smell (hyperosmia); fumbles; falls; wide-based gait.

Peripheral: Dysesthesias; pain; fasciculations; hyperreflexia; hypersensitivity.

Autonomic: Adrenal exhaustion; elevated corticosteroid levels; lid lag; decreased blood pressure; poor response to postural change; difficulty swallowing; intestinal stasis; incomplete voiding on urination.

May carry labels such as peripheral (and/or cranial) neuritis or neuropathy; degenerative neurological diseases like MS, ALS, ADHD; Parkinson's disease; dementia; thought or mood disorders; or suicide.

GASTROINTESTINAL
Loss of symbionts that aid digestion, produce nutrients, and protect the gut from toxins, allergens, and pathogens; overgrowth of organisms that produce toxins,

bloating, food cravings, and alternating constipation and diarrhea; aggravation by antibiotic use, poor inoculation in infancy, and poor replenishment by soils; inflammation of gut lining.

May carry labels such as gastritis, reflux (GERD), functional/irritable bowel syndrome, food intolerances; nutrient deficiencies, food or systemic allergies with rash and asthma, yeast overgrowth, or leaky bowel syndrome.

IMMUNE SYSTEM & ALLERGY

Asthma: food allergies; leaky bowel with circulating immune complexes—pruritic rash, bronchospasm, changes in T-cell fractions; low WBC count.

May carry labels such as asthma, allergies, or immune dysfunction.

MUSCULOSKELETAL SYSTEM

Myalgias, arthralgias, myofascial tenderness (trigger points); exercise intolerance due to poisons blocking electrotransport chain, with increased fat mobilization that increases poisons.

May carry label such as mitochondrial dysfunction (mito.)

OTHER

Night sweats; "flu"; nausea; headache; loss of alertness; sleep disturbances; episodic and diurnal flares; recurrent vaginitis due to GI yeast overgrowth; urinary tract infections secondary to microbiome degradation or poor voiding; mild hypothyroidism; hypoglycemic episodes; obesity due to avoidance of catabolism and toxin release; mouth ulcers; rhinitis; sinus headaches; gingivitis; and gingival recession.

May carry labels such as ME, CFS, CFIDS, FM, MCS, EHS, mental Illness, or neurotoxicity.

human-caused illnesses requires time, contemplation, courage, and a gradual increase in awareness and perspective. Those who learn from life rather than from databases and experts will find it easiest to comprehend emerging epidemics as illnesses of the body of life that affect the bodies of habitats, species, and individuals. During the Iron Age, Hippocrates wrote of the impact of agriculture and locale on disease in *Ancient Medicine* and in *Airs, Waters and Places.* We can remember much lost wisdom by reading medical history, while also appreciating the advantages that have come with every era.

In clinical medicine, doctors can open their minds and consider causal models of illnesses related to environmental poisoning and degradation. They may also contemplate the effects of occupational exposures to agricultural chemicals, as well as of exposures to items on the red list of chemicals prohibited by the Living Building Challenge (a green building paradigm and sustainable design framework that visualizes the ideal for the emerging built environment).

Clinicians who consider chronic poisoning as a possibility in their patients can: include it in their differential diagnoses, increase their diagnostic index of suspicion prudently and appropriately, and try cure cautiously in cases of Chronic Fatigue Syndrome (CFS), Fibromyalgia (FM), Attention Deficit/Hyperactivity Disorder (ADHD), chronic Lyme Disease, Multiple Chemical Sensitivity (MCS), Electromagnetic Hypersensitivity, (EHS), Myalgic Encephalomyelitis (ME), Parkinson's Disease, Amyotrophic Lateral Sclerosis (ALS), and other ailments that may be caused or worsened by chronic preventable chemical and non-ionizing radiation exposure.

In sum, my cure is to stop ingesting, inhaling, and absorbing poisons and irritants, and to avoid non-ionizing radiation. For a more in-depth view, ask your doctor, or find a doctor familiar with the website LivingFutureMedicine.com

It used to be said that he who knows syphilis knows medicine; and then that he who knows AIDS knows medicine. At this moment in history, it can reasonably be said that she who knows Alderman syndrome (chronic ambient poisoning) knows medicine.

CHAPTER EIGHT

Observing Life: Excerpts

T HOSE WHO HAVE HAD TO PRACTICE the science of everyday life as a way of pursuing personal cure will understand the need to observe its nitty-gritty details over and over again for a long period of time. This kind of focused attention to a deep and broad collection of raw data is required to make general statements that constitute information, stories that create meaning, or the experiential wisdom to pattern care or cure. In this chapter, I share some of my daily struggles with discovery to prepare you for what it may be like.

The daily life of medical detection is—to put it bluntly—a grinding bore. It's a matter of repeating observations indefinitely. It's taking a full-time interest in innards and their irritants. Your conversation may become like the "organ recital" of the elderly that expands to fill conversation and bears little resemblance to daytime hospital soap operas or prime time medical dramas. Next to work in the operating room, emergency room, or Intensive care unit, it's as exciting as watching the cracks on the sidewalk so as to not step on them. Observation of this kind is certainly not integrative, transformational, or inspirational. That comes later, when you define obstacles and turn them into opportunities for comprehension and creativity.

Late August, 2017: Fire Season in Southern Oregon

After a wet and snowy winter when I wasn't sure I could drive to the grocery store, the hot summer turned the western side of the continental divide into a tinderbox. The guys on the construction crew, who were remodeling my newly-purchased house to make it safer for me, got the mini-split installed just in time. This ductless heating, cooling, and air filtration system could bring the daytime temperature well below one hundred degrees inside, and remove the smoke too. Although still toxic, I was highly motivated to give this new electrical cooling system a try.

The smoke clouds, when they came, were so thick I couldn't see across the street. I had a mask—the "I can breathe" mask developed for the Beijing Olympics—but it wasn't good enough. I had to stay indoors a lot. That was prudent anyway, as the smoke smelled toxic, perhaps from the weather inversions that trapped I-5 exhaust in the valley, or from appliances, heavy equipment, or other potentially toxic materials vaporized with the homes and lands caught in extremely high-temperature fires. I thought of the studies of lung diseases worsened by Mount St. Helens when it erupted in the 1980s. I also thought about air pollution emergencies, which could precipitate breathing problems—even death—and felt this smoke sinister.

I turned on my new mini-split and went to sleep in my bedroom, which had been the least toxic room in the house. I woke up feeling poorly. I became more and more toxic. Was I breathing the toxins, or were they going right through me? I wasn't sure. I realized that while the cooling unit was way down the hall, the "line set" that fed it included a copper pipe, coolant and 240-volt line that ran from the condenser outside, past the electrical box, under the floor, up through the bedroom closet, and then through the dining room ceiling to the mini-split unit. I seemed to feel all of it. We would have to take this mitigation experiment to the next level.

In the meantime, I would have to cut the power to see if I could get some relief. When the breaker switch went off, I felt an immediate effect. It was a strange set of symptoms: chills, not rigors, more like the end of a sharp hot flash; and my thoughts stopped skipping tracks as they had been since going to bed the night before, even in dreams. I also had a headache, nausea, and a dark, heavy, blank feeling. It was a clear demonstration that the toxicity was whole-body—something one may be most aware of when an intense "dirty" field cuts out abruptly.

~

How ambivalent I feel when I'm talking about my illness to somebody else! Part of me wants others to know everything, and part of my toxicity is to prattle. The heart of me yearns to have an intelligent conversation about what is happening within that will help me think it through, or at least to have someone who would bear witness to what I'm learning. I am alone in this, holding a heavy burden of knowledge that no one will bear with me. Which is another reason I talk and talk, like Cassandra, trying to warn anyone who will listen.

October 2017

One of the not-so-great aspects of life in Ashland is that it's the most allergenic place in the country—according to my allergist. Last spring, there were times when I could only walk a couple of blocks as compared to the usual mile or two, even though I was now taking inhaled steroids and albuterol year-round. When a friend suggested allergy shots, I got a referral to an allergist who found skin tests positive for the usual local suspects: California black oak, beech, and alder trees, and four grasses. I don't get itchy eyes, runny nose, or sneezing very often; my most frequent reaction is to have the smallest airways in my lungs clamp down—and to cough up thick sputum.

I started allergy shots, but developed a cold with airway hyper-reactivity, and had to stop and take a short course of prednisone. I don't know how people tolerate that. Now I'm starting the shots again. About twenty-four hours after the first shot, I had a sick day with flu-like feelings. I had to lie down. I lost a day of work. I crossed my fingers that I'd be able to continue and be desensitized by spring. I can't take antihistamines because they aggravate my neurotoxicity, and I can't buy anything else here that might work.

End of November 2017

My husband and kids were here for Thanksgiving. We had a good family visit, but I overdid things. I had a tablespoon of liquor every day, and one drink with a generous shot of brandy in it. I went out to restaurants with relatively high levels of non-ionizing radiation. I was in the car a lot, went to movies, and generally did much more than usual.

The undercurrents of family dynamics also got me down. For example, my husband, who can't bear to be separated from his electronic devices, was sneaking his phone under the covers. I called him on it, and he got angry. He started to ridicule me and encouraged our children to do the same. None of them has read what I've written. My husband views me as a psychiatric case and alternately humors me, tests me with hidden devices, or ridicules me and tells everyone we know that I'm crazy. They believe him. In other words, the more I need his consideration, the more he scapegoats me and isolates me from family and friends.

When they left, I was tired, frightened, and depressed. For the first time I could remember, I felt that I had no reason to live, and no reason to work. What difference could I make? Why should I try? Look how those closest to me behaved. They didn't want to visit me in Ashland. The kids wanted to be in the city; my husband wanted to be at work.

Now I am seriously suicidal. Empty of light. Without hope. Last year I had nowhere to go, no way to connect with people who put their cellphones first—and who learn from pop culture that I must be crazy and deserve shunning. I could end up that way again. I could be there now.

December 2017

My feet have started to hurt and to cramp. This happened last year, too. My toes move spontaneously; my second right toe beats gently back and forth like a metronome. I give away my hard-bottomed hiking boots because my feet hurt. I feel as if the floor is vibrating. I can't sit for any period of time without my feet going numb. I stand on a pillow to write.

Last year, I had been able to trace the problem to my earthing sheet, which I placed across the bottom of the bed under my heels. Shot through with a copper mesh, it could be plugged into the grounding receptacle of an electrical outlet and so generate a field that was close to that of the Earth whereon our species evolved—or that was the idea. It was close to electrically neutral if there were no errors in wiring, no sources of dirty electricity—such as a wireless monitor—*and* nothing drawing power from the circuit. When I stopped using it as directed, my feet returned almost to normal.

This time, I think the allergy shots awakened my immune system. My lung and gut problems, and my incipient peripheral neuropathy, must have an immune component. I'll have to stop the shots. What will I do?

One good thing about my present predicament is that I'm having one or many loose stools every day. Previously, I spent a lot of time worrying about constipation. Almost every day, in fact. But not now! I am officially no longer full of shit.

∼

I am trying to rally. I can help myself. I can ask for help. I am trying not to feel like a giraffe who doesn't belong anywhere near here. I am trying not to miss the interfaith community in Seattle. At least I can carry them in my heart.

I stop the sips of alcohol. I stay in the house or walk in the woods as much as possible. I confide in a neighbor who is kind to me. Two friends in faraway cities call. My nurse practitioner ups my antidepressant dose and refers me to a neurologist. I stop the shots and put myself on ibuprofen.

Still, it is a dark time. My long-time editor has cancer. My cowriter and other collaborators are unhappy with me. My Jewish-Yule dinner fails to attract guests.

But then my daughter comes to visit. She cooks for me, and tries mountain bike riding—makes a real effort to like visiting. I begin to recover my meaning and purpose. Her love soaks into me, restores me.

～

I get headaches from changes in the electromagnetic field, not from the intensity per se. Going from a more normal electromagnetic field to a less normal one, and back again, is quite jostling. Getting on a cell phone is abnormal in one way, walking under a mini-split unit in another, sleeping on the earthing sheet in a different way again—perhaps because it is uniform. Going from one to the other is problematic.

I've slept with the earthing sheet right under the back of my head. This causes brain fog, too. A brighter-feeling one, but still fuzzy. The brain is meant to generate its own unimaginably complex milieu. A man in town built a greenhouse addition for this condition so that he can sleep on the ground, and so support the function of his brain the way it evolved.

～

I'm getting more symptoms of fibromyalgia. I've heard of the crossover between CFS and fibromyalgia, but have never felt the latter so clearly before. I have pain in my tendons and ligaments, and what feels like a kind of arthritis. It's not just my feet; it's also my wrists. I thought it was because I was writing a lot … but I actually haven't been writing a lot.

～

I am accumulating fat again. Now that I'm walking less, my metabolism is subsiding and my overall health is slipping.

I'm damned if I do walk, and damned if I don't. The intangible body that is generated by my flesh when I do walk is very important for my functioning and well-being. That *is* my body, really, the important part of it; the functionality of it. And so, when I can walk in the woods again, I'll be able to boost my vitality—but my feet still hurt too much, and I have to be patient.

The weather is favorable this winter: often clear and sunny, and mild. But the setbacks make it difficult to enjoy it. The dark force of my immune system is inflaming my body. I may have to take the prednisone, but first I'll cut out black tea, dairy, wheat, and the things that seem to be irritating my gut and microbiome in the absence of exercise. And try to walk a little more each day.

～

Clinicians are situationally brave. They are trained to condition themselves completely to the environment in which they're working as fast and as seamlessly as possible to smooth the workings of the social medical machine. You can get so good at it that you have no idea what's going on outside the doors of the hospital.

And you can be very brave *in* the hospital, while not being very brave outside of it.

～

Receiving and integrating, or listening and integrating, with listening including a spiritual dimension: This is what brought me back around to the recognition that our bodies are antennae. Each one of us is an antenna and a conductor. I think that's a critical concept. Once you get that the nervous system is an antenna that picks up the radiation emitted by our electric and electronic devices, you can grasp how it might give you migraines, depression, epilepsy, "chronic fatigue," psychosis, fibromyalgia, or whatever it may be.

It's strange that despite the fact we know strobes can trigger epilepsy, that tasers can be dangerous, that electro-convulsive therapy can do great harm—and that electromyography, electrocardiography, and electroencephalography give us useful information about the body—people can still imagine that the body is impervious to non-ionizing radiation. We view radiation in the electromagnetic range through a perceptual filter that is peculiar at best. It seems that when Benjamin Franklin did his experiment with electricity and invented the lightning rod, it helped so much in preventing house fires that we put electricity into a safe and trusted box. But we have left it there; we have been oblivious, and overconfident, ever since.

And now we've gone from having a single lightbulb in the ceiling of dining room to having extraordinary light pollution that baffles our habitats, with our electricity use consuming power as if there were no tomorrow. And perhaps ensuring that there is none.

We've gone from heated controversy about microwave ovens to disseminating cell phones, wi-fi, and microwave towers that turn the whole planet into a microwave oven! Some say that if it is too weak to cook our brains, it isn't a problem. How we misuse our assumptions! As archaeologists put it, absence of evidence is not evidence of absence.

What if the effects are worse than that? What if radiation causes dark urban fantasies and rural shootings? Will we be so addicted to our devices, and so unable to see the problem, that we'll be unable to change?

～

I go to see the neurologist. He is kind. He finds, in keeping with my symptoms, that my nerve conduction velocities are a little lower on the right than on the left, but the nerves in both legs are still in the normal range. He reassures me by saying that I'll be a hundred years old before it gets so bad as to require an intervention like amputation—which is a polite way of saying that I'll die of something else before getting serious peripheral neuropathy. That is a great relief. When I ask what the treatment would be if it became abnormal, he says, "None." It would be untreatable. I decide to stick with my efforts to realize preventive cure, which means that I may have to leave the Rogue Valley.

October 2018

I go out to eat at a new restaurant that advertises non-GMO, organic ethnic food. The menu items include traditional pork dishes and new-fangled vegetarian or vegan ones. When I ask about how they source the food, I recognize it as cheap rather than safe. I order it anyway. I have been wondering whether I may have recovered some tolerance, so I experiment.

I regret it that night when I wake up in pain, and the next day when I feel sick. I realize that this is my chance to observe a single poisoning event. My symptoms linger for nine days. I do not develop the neuritis, but my thinking is fuzzy and I have trouble with the spatial task of assembling a jigsaw puzzle. I don't know how I managed to live through a more intense state for fifteen years; perhaps because my children were small and I did not want to leave them.

During this time, I recognize that I have in general recovered enough that the earthing sheet now does more harm than good. This confirms the expectation that I will be pursuing medical detection for this illness and cure for the rest of my life.

November 2018

I spend two hours on the computer with a phone "hotspot" and—by mistake—with the microwave of the computer wi-fi on. I am attempting to use my computer once a week in order to accomplish tasks that are difficult to do without it. I seemed to be fine the first few times, but I feel this and know that I must cease to avoid losing what health I have managed to regain over the last six years.

After the exposure on Day One, I get up on Day Two feeling as if I have a hangover. I'm cranky, my mind is full of complaints; I'm achy, slow and heavy, and the top and back of my head pain me. I amble around my home, which helps, but it makes my feet tingle.

On Day Three, I put date pits in my oatmeal and loose tea leaves in my cup of hot water. My tremor is such that when I try to use a pot, much of the water ends up on the counter as I pour it through the tea caddy. I feel back to baseline, but I'm not. Thoughts that ran through my had last year and that made me feel distant from myself are back. I'll try to regain some normality with a hike.

∼

Who knows what I will have to learn the hard way next time? I can only hope that I will find my way to a family or a community who will want to catch me the next time I fall.

CHAPTER NINE

Climate Change Refugee

———

THE LATE SPRING OF 2018 brought me to a new level of recovery. A year earlier I had recovered coincidence, and could tell that my circadian rhythms and my waking and dreaming perceptions were normalizing. This allergy season, without the shots, I have been able to enjoy the trails near my home, many of which pass through the meticulously maintained watershed above town. After it suffered the controlled burns of early spring, I was able to hike for two hours in the evening several times a week. Without my noticing it, my mind became clearer. When it came time to proof my books, I identified problems that I couldn't see before, and wanted the chance to bring them up a notch. My recovery became an upward spiral. My perpetual crucifixion and resurrection left the realm of tangible pain and suffering and problem-solving and rose to a realm in which I could attempt to embody wise action in the world. I looked forward to being able to conform.

And then smoke season began. It came a month early, on the fourth of July, when a careless human ignited the forest south of the Oregon border, in California. Others began soon after, and we were once again blanketed in smoke and looking ahead to a four-month heavy smoke season. From my front window I saw a red ball of sun casting indistinct salmon-colored shadows through downy gray air. When I drove down the hill past the closest access to the Pacific Crest Trail, hoping to glimpse the rock-tipped panorama of the Rogue Valley below, I saw only a wall of white smog. What had been figuratively breathtaking was now literally so. Over ensuing weeks, I saw blue in the heavens now and then, and one weekend was able to go outside without a mask.

Hiking was out of the question due to the choking smoke; I went to the YMCA. My home remained the one place that my lungs and mind could both be safe. As the smoke settled in and the heat increased, I had to turn on the ductless cooling and air filtration system while I was out of the house. And so my world got smaller but remained safe enough to allow me to continue my activities. But then the YMCA filled with smoke, and my mask was not enough. I had to stay at home with the cooling system on. Knowing that I could not stay for the three or more months of smoke season that remained, I then fled in search of a place in nature with clean air, food, and water free of radiation.

August 2018: Life Poses a Question

Discovery is chasing me now. As Dr. Viktor Frankl taught after his experience in the death camps, it is meaning and purpose that keep us alive, the meaning and purpose that we create in response to the questions that life asks us. For me, these are big ones like: what can doctors do to save the body of our species and the body of life—both of which our species now controls—from the sixth extinction that will soon be irreversible? Life also poses constant small questions like: what can I eat now without poisoning my beleaguered body?

Today I hold a beautifully presented chocolate bar in my hand. It is contained in an elegant cardstock cover lined with foil. The beauty shot on the back shows a woman who claims to be doing everything possible to create sustainable products. This one includes black Hawaiian salt, and it is GMO-free but not organic. For years people have asked me questions that at times, years later, help clarify my understanding. One is whether GMO foods are a problem for me. I have been saying no because I could not see how such a diverse set of processes could have the same effects or how any of them might poison me.

I know about the poison cocktail that has sickened me for decades. I know that when Rachel Carson wrote *Silent Spring*, the pervasive wishful thinking that problems like ambient DDT poisoning could be fixed one molecule at a time had led to an ineffectual response. I know that over-complicating a problem obscures its causes and consequences and blocks prevention. I know that organic farming and biomass preservation—to the extent possible with today's unprecedented high minimum night time temperatures—may be solutions.

On the other hand, I also know that during the time frame of my illness, the simultaneous overuse by industrial farmers of organophosphorus, Bt-producing corn, and highly concentrated crop derivatives have been impacting all kinds of processed foods—such as chocolate bars. I also know that high levels of Bt are turning up in umbilical cord blood, and that it may be a particularly bad actor in human health now and into the future.

I have been intending to experiment with non-GMO foods, but being alone in the world means that I need to have a clear head. I have been waiting for a time when I could afford a serious setback. And now, thanks to my daughter who is driving us eastward, things are going well, and I have almost escaped my latest emergency in reasonably good shape. Though there is no truly safe place for me to go, and I am having the occasional EMF-caused headache, I have a delicious experiment in hand and hope that it will be a safe bet because I bought it at the excellent food co-op in Moab, Utah.

I take a bite. I take a few more bites. And then I devour what remains, wincing at my recklessness before I forget all about the experiment and simply enjoy the fact that I have a treat. After a period of hypnosis by the sagebrush-covered scenery of Western Colorado, I realize that nothing happened. Nothing happens at night either.

$\sim$

I am haunted by the skeletons of trees that we see on our drive through Rocky Mountain National Park. In the early 1980s, when I lived in Denver and hiked and snowshoed in the Rocky Mountains, I knew about the pine beetle. More recently, I heard that it had spread. Now, at an interpretive panel on the side of Trail Ridge Road, I see a map of the present extent of beetle damage. The entire Pacific watershed of North America, every still-forested habitat west of the Continental Divide, appears to be infected.

This is the only place in the park where I see mention of the fact that the beetle is not the enemy. The beetle is only the scapegoat. The culprit is tree stress due to heat and drought, which is caused by our species' destruction, consumption, and poisoning of the body of life that creates our climate—especially the coastal forests critical to cloud formation. According to an article in the newspaper, it is the rising of mean daily low temperatures that is harming the last of the wild habitats in the West. The territory of the pine beetle is set to become a new Sahara. And the death of life is well under way.

I am crushed. My vision of habitat restoration and integration as a means to prevent human extinction goes up in flames. I remember attending a retreat some years ago at which an academic physicist got up and cried into the microphone about the redwoods around his campus, how sensitive they were to temperature, how they would be gone in twenty years. How few were aware, how few wanted to know or acknowledge the death on the horizon.

I was listening to him, feeling with him, and losing faith in our almost-glorious species and its inadvertent homicide-suicide plan. We are better at denying, catastrophizing, whining, and demonizing than we are at rolling up our sleeves and cleaning up our mess—even when we are in grave peril. References to Muggles and zombies are apt. How will I keep my expectations high enough to continue fighting for the species and at the same time low enough for each person I know who has lost the ability to listen and comprehend?

Right now my hopes are reduced to finding a place where the air, water, food, and electromagnetic milieu will be safe for a while. I'm glad that my daughter got to see the body of life, and that I, at least, am doing what little I can to save it.

CHAPTER TEN

New Vision

_____

THE GREATEST THREAT TO HUMAN HEALTH is the modern way of life that is causing extinction. According to Elisabeth Kolbert's *The Sixth Extinction* and other resources, we may have a hundred years to mitigate and reverse our destruction before it dooms our species and all others. Given the present burning of temperature-sensitive habitats, we may have much less. What are doctors doing to prevent this catastrophe? Too little. The way we are going, we are saving the patient and losing the species. We are caring for the child and abetting the loss of her future. We are serving the desires of a society that needs the resilience of a profession that has transformed with every era. It is time to let go of modernity and to embrace and evolve the emerging paradigm that may allow us to engage deep biological time.

So. How do we get from our present absorption in virtual reality that is disconnected from our present biological reality and its escalating catastrophes (Point A) to a positive engagement with life on earth that synergizes with the body of life and that cares for and cures humans in context (Point B)? In other words, how do we choose life? How do we recognize our earthly Eden for the shared treasure that it is?

Let's look at some aspects of the new paradigm proposed by Evolve Medicine, the not-for-profit think-tank that I am founding to alter our frames and constructs so that we can approach patients as integral to life on earth. Let's try and appreciate and enhance what remains of the last 300 million years of evolution rather than settling for leaving the Earth to cockroaches and similarly simple and resilient survivors. The idea is to transform modern medicine into a means of creating a living future in which humans cooperate with life and so learn to survive and thrive. The time to do it is now, when success may still be possible.

Care Contextualized. The focal point of my meaning and purpose—the thing that keeps me alive the way Viktor Frankl's book kept him alive through the *Shoah*—is imagining what it would be like to take the first few steps through the looking glass into emerging medicine. I picture a care team with a doctor trained in medical detection; a bodyworker who embodies and shares care; a counselor for putting the past to rest and for family engagement; and a habitat restorer and integrator. Together the team would assist the patient with chronic illness of no known cause; they would ease the patient's suffering and advise her in creating and adapting a plan for self-care integrated with care for the species, habitat, and body of life.

The clinic would be off the grid in every respect. It would also be residential, like a sanatorium, and located on a large parcel of land in need of gentle restoration to return it to the wild state. If near sufficient and sustainable supplies of water, it would be irrigated and protected from fire until temperatures fall. Housed in a living building surrounded by permaculture, the facility would be on land purchased by retirees as their place of residence. It would serve for end of life care, and would self-fund through patient fees, teaching, and food production. Once up and running, foundation grant money would support a fellowship program in emerging paradigm medicine for newly board-certified physicians, and another for retiring physicians who are transitioning to medical elderhood.

In this vision, doctors live forward as explorers of the universe of the body, knowing that they are well-equipped to do this work and that new knowledge is required in real time without filtration through the old academic model—or any centralized top-down modern system. In this vision, the compassion movement catalyzed by religious scholar Karen Armstrong's TED award overtakes the hunger for raw data and dazzling—but disappointing and destructive—technologies that look amazing but over-consume resources and lead to overdiagnosis. In this vision, we spend the resources we can gather while adding to the future of life, and no more. We nurture life instead of taking it. We live and learn to live better as we are evolved to do in order to deserve descendants.

Let's take a closer look at a few aspects of this dream.

Living the Science of Everyday Life. To reveal the way that chronic ambient poisoning affects humans, we must start with the assumption that everyone is different, and that there will be no "magic bullet" in the form of one or a few causative poisons or susceptibility genes. Any ailment that has not already caused one or more irreversible (final common pathway) anatomical diseases can be investigated by a patient supported by a doctor—or by a doctor-patient—as described in this book.

The only new characteristic of this use of the N-of-1 method is that it addresses prevention and cure as one. In other words, it addresses ailments closer to the beginning of the causal web. Look around you: your modern way of life is the source of death. As in every era, what you don't know—or don't want to know—can and will kill our species and our context as well.

Habitat Transition and Restoration. At this point in late modernity, life is in need of intensive care. The body of humanity is caching organic poisons in its tissues and heavy metals in its bones in many of the habitats on which the biosphere relies. At this time, it is impossible to view human fertility in the old way, or to view the body of life as we have done previously. We have done too much damage.

But solutions to these problems are already forming as emerging paradigms. These support our species in withdrawing from thoughtless destruction and consumption, and in rehabilitating and regenerating the body of humanity as the body of life. This change is ready to inspire evolution in allopathic views, definitions, and practices.

For example, you might view fertility as increasing life on Earth by adopting habitats that you heat-transition and restore, perhaps with the aid of desalination and irrigation and perhaps by integrating our species into them as carers. You might view infertility as a gateway to exploring ways of nurturing new life in the body of life and as many of its evolved aspects as possible, including you. That would take each of us acting according to our abilities and opportunities—and prioritizing the forests that are the lungs of the body of life, and that are fast disappearing.

Allopathy as Field Biology. We are a species. We belong to other species. No walls can obliterate our human dependence on, and interdependence with, the other species that comprise our habitats and the body of life. To care for each human being and for the body of humanity, you recognize all as being integral members of the sacred body of life—and the need to care for all lives as one. Facing the choice between killing the future of life on Earth or taking the body of life as a patient and caring for and curing it, you can choose life as we could know it. As others have pointed out, it is the eleventh hour—but it is never too late to do the right thing in good faith. The practical periphery can do this; the virtual center may be too disconnected from its living habitats to offer aid.

When you look back to the beginning of the end of late modernity, you see that efforts to turn medicine into science forced clinical science into a narrow view of life dominated by molecular science, statistics, and data processing. Through programs such as MSTP (medical science training program), young physicians of my generation were taught to look down on field biology and clinical sciences and to lionize those who believed that imaging could reveal everything of importance, if only the picture were sharp enough. These methods have certainly yielded gifts of understanding, and may continue to have value if we find a way to put them into perspective. That perspective will come from taking the body of life as our patient, and grounding our care in the human scale and in the biosphere. In doing so, we can ground medicine in eco-centric field biology and learn to survive and thrive in vivo.

If you look at the body of humanity from the perspective of the body of life, you can see allopathy as just another of the field sciences, and thus open new kinds of collaboration. For example, veterinarians could identify domesticated animals whose milk does not—for whatever reason—hold or transmit poisons, and local agronomists might inform doctors as to which soils and foods are poison-free, or may become so with care. With such collaborators, we can update the public health regulations that have entrapped us so that they serve the future of life.

When you are well, the illusion of control can lead you to rationalize the management of medicine as a perfectible manufacturing process or abstract pursuit of arbitrary ideas about anatomical, genetic, robotic, or off-world perfection. When you get sick, you may have to improvise, and emergence can support that. And while trust supports emergence, blind trust leads to fantastic cloud castles such as notions of personal immortality of the kind that inevitably lead to disillusionment.

Gardens Wild and Tame. We literally breathe and drink wilderness. Without it, the naturally-filtered sweet water and plant-produced oxygen on which we depend could not exist. No human effort to replace nature could do these things, but simple acceptance and solicitous care of creation can. You and I are children of a wild mother that has fed us and will continue to do so, if we choose survival over extinction. And while we will change her body as we grow and develop, we can cultivate her wilds as well as sustainable proportions of local arable and pastureland—whatever those may turn out to be.

When we cultivate the thin living skin of the Earth as a wild and tame garden that guides us, there will be no human-created wastelands, no city walls to separate the body of humanity from the body of life. Megalomaniacal millennial plans, and their catastrophic consequences, serve as cautionary tales about concretizing and fixing ideas and planning from the dissociated center. Even now, bioarcheology is turning the whole of the human record into an open book filled with inspiring tales of continuation, adaptation, and transformation.

Land for Life's Sake. Forest habitats don't grow by rehabilitating or regenerating branches; they multiply generously and, when allowed to do so, extend across the terrain and mature as they have evolved to do—so long as either the conditions that supported their evolution continue or the species that changed those conditions takes responsibility for the consequences to creation. While extinction can spread through history and conclude in a lifetime, evolution transpires over time periods so great as to elude embodied comprehension. Understanding evolution requires well-grounded, empirical constructs that correspond to material evidence. We sometimes lionize and adore our results, including them in the modern theology that we call science—but this misleads and mystifies us. Science is a tool kit, and what we learn by using these tools is no more than our wits allow, and these have the capacity to create an evolving guide to choosing life and creating a living future for well-grounded, synchronous minds.

Land use is an expression of delicate and sometimes fanciful human processes. It may seem right and inevitable, *until it teaches us to be horrified by the inadvertent harm we are doing*—harm which is quite possibly fatal. We are already extinguishing the sources of oxygen in the sea, as well as those on land that are being replaced by human-centric modern structures inspired by the stony bones of civilizations that ended in desertification.

Emerging land use therefore departs from the hugely destructive habits of late modernism. It abjures thoughtless destruction and consumption habits bequeathed to us by forebears who also left us surviving centers of life that may still regenerate—but only if we turn to habitat restoration, transition, and integration.

The Habitat of the Individual. The epidemics due to land consumption, modern poisoning, and medical neglect of the body of life can be solved with the foundation of residential habitat restoration clinics and communities. Experimental and voluntary, these would enable self-guided caregivers and curers to come together to care for the body of life with and through the bodies of individuals and their local habitats. With teams that care for both the tangible and intangible, and networks of consultants who offer relevant knowledge and skills, such communities could pattern habitat integration, green schools, the new economy, emerging fertility, and other creative endeavors through which multiple local experiments could come together to form a new global paradigm (see the Fertility and Restoration series).

It's certainly worth a try. If we become worthy caretakers of life, we may survive through a long, cyclical metamorphosis the likes of which none of us can foresee now.

My dream, then, is to become a doctor of the species in its living context. A doctor of life. That would be marvelous indeed. And, dare I say it? It could be fun, inspiring, and engaging! Compelling. And we could—through the catalysis of medical renewal—deserve the Eden that is our heritage, and also the posterity that will care for it.

Acknowledgements

I owe my faith in humanity to those peers and mentors who engage the unknown as a source of sacred and inchoate new knowledge to be perceived and brought to light for the betterment of the world: particularly Michael Goodman, Ronald Perline, Professor Peter Meier, and Professor Monte Lloyd. I owe my patterning for discovery to those teachers who shared ideas and methods for inviting or embodying new knowledge: Rev. Cynthia Bourgeault, Imam Jamal Rahman, Rabbi Zalman Schachter-Shalomi, Rev. Matthew Fox, Geshe Kelsang Gyatso, Mantak Chia, Phabongkha Rinpoche, Sakya Monastery, and most of all Rabbi Ted Falcon.

I owe a deep debt of gratitude to: the University of Chicago method of free and open exchange of ideas; investigators who mentored me in laboratory sciences including C. N. Yang and Lucia Rothman-Denes; past physicians who gave their lives to advance the profession, especially Semmelweis and Dr. Howard Taylor Ricketts, whose portrait hung at the end of a hallway in the Pritzker School of Medicine; those mentors who taught me about medical detection and population medicine, especially Dr. Pierce Gardner, Drs. Tom Vernon and Ellen Mangione, Drs. Jose Cordero and David Swanson; Bill Foege and his colleagues for showing that humans can cure the species; and most of all Dr. Buchanan, master of the teaching anecdote, and his lineage of Edinburgh-trained doctors that trace back to the Scottish Enlightenment, when inspired physicians intervened and began to try for cure.

I am similarly indebted to those who are leading the present sea change in other fields, and who taught me about the emerging paradigm, especially: field biologists Joe Hutto and Janine Benyus through their TED talks; the New Hassids and New Monastics in religion and theology, and other unitive thinkers presently doing retreats; the developers of the seven petal living building paradigm and the Bullitt Center, especially Bob Hull and Mike Jobes; and Hammer-in-Hand, TC Legend Homes, and Anne Raab.

A number of teachers and colleagues helped me to see medicine from a psychological or anthropologic perspective, to see the errors and arbitrary constructs that limit and warp medical judgement, and to avoid mindless conformity to the herd mentality: Arthur Elstern; Amos Tversky and David Kahneman; the Society for Medical Decision Making; Dr. Alvan Feinstein; Ron LaPorte; Lorna Moore; in the clinic setting, Drs. Mond and Shapiro; and student Nancy Gegen.

Equally instrumental in the development of my perspective as a physician were those who acquainted me with medicine in various populations: Dr. Joel Mason and his father, who arranged a summer externship at St. Vincent's Hospital in New York; Dr. Joel Silversten and colleagues in Nairobi for the medical student rotation at Kenyatta National Hospital; Dr. Pekka Puska of the International Epidemiology Association meetings in Helsinki and Joensuu; and my husband for taking me to many national and international diabetes meetings. I would also like to thank Howard Nagatani and my other Sansei friends and the Holocaust survivors who inspired me to go on when I thought I couldn't, especially the Sperlings, Jellineks, Philip Maisel, and also Victor and Elly Frankl.

Last but not least I thank my parents for teaching me to respect all people and to value education and culture over money and possessions, and thank Chansonette Beck, Ann DiSalvo, Deidre Krupp, and Deborah Mokma for book development and editing; and Chris Molé for book design.

About the Author

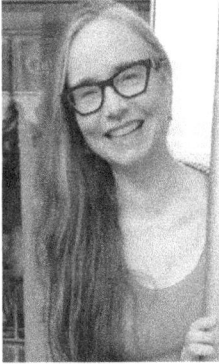

BETH ALDERMAN, MD, MPH earned her AB and MD degrees from the University of Chicago and her MPH from the University of Washington. After Board Certification in Preventive Medicine and Public Health, she took a faculty position in the University of Colorado Medical School Department of Preventive Medicine, Biometrics, and Medical Informatics, where she did population-based epidemiological studies of adverse reproductive outcomes and methodological studies in clinical epidemiology. In her next faculty position at the University of Washington School of Public Health, she focused on risk factors for birth defects.

In 1996, she fell ill with the mysterious new plague and was given the provisional diagnosis "chronic fatigue syndrome". She has spent her time since studying her own case and pondering the reasons that her beloved profession failed her so completely. Fortunately, she discovered her cure, which may be of use to others suffering from one or more of the emerging epidemics affecting humans, their habitats, and life on earth.

For more about and from the author, see the following websites:

BethAldermanMD.com — *Free Information for all readers*
DoctorsOfLife.com — *For care and cure of all lives as one*
LivingFutureBooks.com — *Publishing Website*

Look for author's books on Amazon.com